The Face Laughs While the Brain Cries

The Face Laughs While the Brain Cries

The Education of a Doctor

Stephen L. Hauser, M.D.

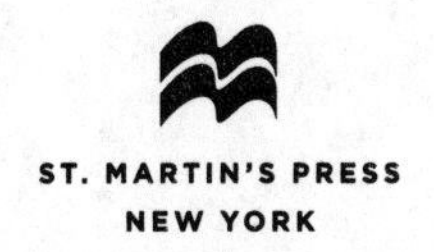

ST. MARTIN'S PRESS
NEW YORK

First published in the United States by St. Martin's Press, an imprint of St. Martin's Publishing Group

www.stmartins.com

Design by Meryl Sussman Levavi

Library of Congress Cataloging-in-Publication Data

Names: Hauser, Stephen L., author.
Title: The face laughs while the brain cries : the education of a doctor / Dr. Stephen L. Hauser, M.D.
Description: First edition. | New York : St. Martin's Press, 2023. | Includes index.
Identifiers: LCCN 2022058228 | ISBN 9781250283894 (hardcover) | ISBN 9781250283900 (ebook)
Subjects: LCSH: Hauser, Stephen L. | Neurologists—Massachusetts—Boston—Biography. | Immunologists—Massachusetts—Boston—Biography. | Multiple sclerosis—Treatment—Anecdotes. | Neuroimmunology—Anecdotes.
Classification: LCC RC339.52.H38 A3 2023 | DDC 616.80092 [B]—dc23/eng/20230125
LC record available at https://lccn.loc.gov/2022058228

First Edition: 2023

10 9 8 7 6 5 4 3 2 1

To Elizabeth

Contents

Author's Note

Names of patients and details of their life stories have been modified just enough to protect their privacy without changing the essential elements or impact of their life-altering illnesses.

I've also taken literary license in recounting the many discussions quoted throughout the book. Some took place more than a half century ago. All represent my best recollection of the actual dialogue that took place, fortified whenever possible by notes, documents, and photos, and by discussions with individuals who were present at the time.

CHAPTER 1

Andrea

Andrea was 27 years old, a beauty queen from Virginia, and a graduate of Harvard Law School. Brilliant, energetic, kind-hearted, and ambitious, she wanted to make a difference, so she chose government service, responding *no thank you* to the big law firms and their promises of early partnerships and seven-figure salaries. She believed in the power of policy and the law to make a positive impact in people's lives; after all, that was why she went to law school in the first place.

She was a rising star, a supernova. Although she was just a few years out of school, her career had already taken off, fueled by a large dose of talent and a dollop of good luck. She had a position in the White House in the early, heady days of the Carter administration. Wonder Woman.

Exactly when the wheels went off the tracks was uncertain, but it was probably no longer than six weeks before we met. It began with changes in behavior that were entirely out of character; she became chatty, seductive, and socially inappropriate. She showed terrible judgment at work. Word soon spread among her colleagues that something was wrong with Andrea. She was seen by a psychiatrist, who suspected a mental disorder, but when counseling failed to reveal a cause and medications didn't help, her family was advised to hospitalize her. But first, the psychiatrist counseled, just to be sure that this wasn't a neurologic problem, maybe Andrea should see a neurologist. Her behavior was so completely out of character, and psychiatric disorders usually don't explode on the scene in this way.

Her frightened parents arranged for Andrea to fly to the Massachusetts General Hospital for a consultation with the renowned neurologist Charles Miller Fisher. Later that day, Fisher told me her story.

"One of the most remarkable cases I've ever seen. Quite astonishing. I heard that she'd be arriving from Washington and told my secretary to have her wait in my office until we finished morning rounds. When I walked in, she was stretched out across the top of my desk, reclining on an elbow, smiling, naked, and dangling a cluster of grapes in her hand. I think that she was reenacting a Roman bacchanal. I spoke to her in a stern voice. 'Please,' I said, 'immediately get off my desk and dress. I'll leave, return in a few minutes, and then let's start again as if this never happened.'"

An injured brain can sometimes direct the body to act inappropriately. Fisher taught us to recognize such changes as a reflection of underlying neurologic disease. Similar to paralysis or loss of speech, abnormal behavior can also help localize where a disease is in the nervous system. The best approach in these situations, he'd say, was to strongly encourage better behavior and hope that less damaged areas of the brain could replace the lost function.

"When I returned, she seemed quite normal, but lacked any awareness that her behavior was odd or that anything was amiss. I couldn't find much else wrong on examination. She was completely oriented, with excellent memory and full command of most facts, and her strength, sensation, coordination, and vision were perfectly normal. I thought that she could safely return to Virginia for close observation until we could learn what was wrong. The cause of her problem would reveal itself over time."

So Andrea was hospitalized in a psychiatric facility in rural Virginia, close to her family's home. Little progress was made. And then, two weeks later, the sky fell in. The medical team was making its morning rounds. When they greeted her, she responded with slurred, mumbled, incoherent vocalizations. She had lost the ability to speak.

Psychiatric diseases sometimes produce speech disturbances. Patients can seem mute; they will use nonsense words, rhyming words, clicking words, or develop a sing-song cadence, but they don't slur or mumble. There was now no doubt that Andrea was suffering from a brain disease, and a terrible one at that.

We carried beepers in those days, little square boxes clipped to our belts that would alert us each time we were needed, telling us to locate a phone and receive a message from the bank of switchboard operators on the top floor of the old hospital building. A late beep usually meant little sleep that night, but no matter, for we were residents, still trainees, and immensely proud to be part of the grand tradition of the august Massachusetts General Hospital. We'd never admit to being tired, or hurried, or sick ourselves. Dedication was taught by example, and our highest goal was to someday practice with the skill of the great ones who taught us. But the beep that brought Andrea into my life was different. It arrived at eight o'clock one morning and came from Dr. Fisher, who never paged me at such an early hour.

"Hello, Steve. Dr. Fisher here," he said. "I need to admit Andrea, the young woman I told you about last month. She seems to have taken a sudden turn for the worse. She's now on her way from Washington and should be here within the hour. Could you see her as soon as she arrives and let me know what you think?"

"Of course," I replied.

When the beeper next went off, it was the message that she'd arrived.

I quickly assigned a few remaining tasks to medical students and interns on our service and ran down to the emergency ward. There, in a small corner room separated from the hallway by only the thinnest of translucent curtains, I saw Andrea for the first time. In a baggy hospital gown, head of bed raised 45 degrees, this young woman, whose life had seemed so full of promise just a few weeks ago, was now bedbound, helpless.

As I pulled the curtains aside and entered the room, she tracked my movements, hyperalert, staring silently. A look of bewilderment was etched on her face. I imagined what she was thinking.

What is happening to me? How can this be possible?

A single tear slowly made its way down her cheek.

Her parents stood helpless at her bedside, overwhelmed, her father's forced smile unable to conceal his agony, her mother gently clasping her hand.

Why her, of all people? Is this somehow our fault?

Nature did not intend it to be this way. Daughter should be tending to parent, not the other way around. They stared at me with a surprised and quizzical look, as if they were wondering about me.

This doctor is no older than our daughter! We flew here, leased a plane, to see Dr. C. Miller Fisher, the great Harvard neurologist, and instead this young resident is taking care of our Andrea. Maybe we should call the head of the hospital. Well, at least he looks professional. Clean white coat, starched button-down shirt, crisply knotted tie, buffed wingtips.

We always looked professional at Massachusetts General Hospital. And what Andrea's parents didn't know was that if you were ill, really ill, a young top-of-game resident with fast reflexes, high octane, and lots of recent experience was your best bet . . . by far.

I began my assessment. The right side of her mouth drooped slightly, and saliva pooled there. Clear signs that the muscles of Andrea's face were no longer receiving proper instructions from the left side of her brain.

Soon, she'll be weaker, I thought, but of more urgent concern was the risk that she'd choke on her secretions or aspirate food into her lungs. *She's critically ill and could suddenly worsen at any time.*

"Hello," I began. "My name is Dr. Steve Hauser. I work with Dr. Fisher."

I reached out to touch her forearm gently, then introduced myself to her folks, shaking hands as we did in those pre-pandemic days. Touching is sometimes the most important thing that a physician can do. A soft touch and a calm voice.

"How are you feeling?"

"Aaar . . . ga."

She tried to sit up to greet me but fell back, torso shaking. My first impression was correct; she had a right hemiparesis (weakness) with ataxia (incoordination). This could be caused by damage at only one discrete place, on the left side of the upper brain stem, just behind the nose. The brain stem is a small area of the brain that connects the overlying cerebral hemispheres with nerve pathways traveling out to the body.

"Is it OK," I asked her, "if your parents stay here with us and I speak with them so that they can help me understand what is happening to you?"

"Ya," she answered, nodding yes.

She understood language, a positive sign. But then an exaggerated yawn, and a burst of explosive laughter. Pseudobulbar palsy, another mark of something wrong at the stem of the brain. A false or inappropriate emotion was a particularly bad sign that signified extensive damage to the emotional circuitry, disconnecting facial expressions from cognitive intent. The face laughs while the brain cries.

I quickly reviewed the records from the psychiatric hospital. The previous evening's report noted that she was unchanged, but her parents told me that her speech had been slurred for at least two days and that yesterday she had difficulty walking, falling over unless she had someone to lean on. Not unusual for medical records to be misleading. So, I knew now that this new problem had come on over a couple of days, on top of the behavioral problem that had first brought her to us.

Andrea's march of symptoms over time wasn't like that of a sudden stroke or a slowly growing brain tumor. She had no fever, and there was no report of headache, ruling out most brain infections. And the damage was asymmetric, more on the right side of the body, so a toxin or a metabolic problem was unlikely since these cause symmetric disturbances. Inflammation was by far the most likely culprit, I thought, but this still could be an unusual virus.

"May I call you Andrea?"

"Ya."

Her speech was limited to a few grunts, and she followed commands poorly. She seemed to be choking.

I turned to her parents.

"Has Andrea ever experienced other neurologic problems," I asked, "either in the distant past or more recently?"

"Yes," her father replied. "A few months ago, she complained of blurred vision on the right."

I looked into her right eye with an ophthalmoscope, a special magnifying lens to peer through the pupil and visualize the retina at the back of the eye. It was clearly swollen. She had inflammation of the nerve that carries visual information and connects the back of the eye to the brain. So, she had damage to at least two places in her nervous system, one on the left side of the upper brain stem and a second in the right optic nerve. Multiple lesions.

This was the key to her problem. Two attacks, separated in time and place, meant that she almost certainly had multiple sclerosis (MS).

Just then, she experienced a brief paroxysm of intense coughing and turned blue, her limbs shaking spasmodically. Her life was in danger, and we needed to move fast.

"Andrea," I said to her, "I think that we should move you to another part of the hospital where we can monitor you more closely, just for a few days. Do you understand what I'm saying? And do you have any questions for me?"

A look of fear, another tear, and a silent shake of her head signifying "no." I glanced at her parents who nodded their assent.

I enlisted the help of two nurses, and after an advance call to the ICU, we transferred her to a stretcher loaded with resuscitation supplies in case of disaster during the transport and raced to the intensive care unit. Here we could manage her ABCs—airway, breathing, and circulation—and because she was young and otherwise healthy, I was hopeful that, once stabilized, she might improve from this catastrophic attack, which had disabled critical life support centers in the brain stem.

"Can you excuse us for a moment and wait in the visitors' room?" I asked her parents, who had followed us to the ICU. They didn't need to see what would happen next.

As soon as they left, I inserted a breathing tube to protect her airway, then a nasogastric tube from her nose to her stomach so she could be fed. There was also an intravenous line for fluids and medications. Several blood tests were needed, mostly to exclude other causes of this catastrophic illness. But by far, the most important diagnostic test would be to examine the cerebrospinal fluid, liquid from the fluid-filled sac that encircles the brain and spinal cord.

For this, I needed to do a spinal tap. I rolled her gently onto her side and, with a nurse's assistance, bent her legs into a fetal position. Then, explaining each step as I went along, not knowing whether she understood me, I sterilized her lower back, carefully inserted the long spinal needle, measured the pressure of the fluid, and withdrew the clear liquid for study.

I hurried down the hall to examine the fluid with a small microscope located in the residents' sleeping quarters. No sign of infection, but numerous white blood cells, clear evidence of inflammation. Results from the key test—measurement of specific immune molecules called oligoclonal bands—wouldn't be available for several days. Oligoclonal bands are abnormal antibodies made by a subset of white blood cells called B lymphocytes, or B cells. Their presence would indicate MS. At the time, we believed that these antibodies were simply markers of the disease and had nothing whatsoever to do with its cause. Overturning this concept would become a central focus of my professional life.

When Andrea's test came back, it was overwhelmingly positive. Her spinal fluid was packed with antibodies, a tsunami of oligoclonal bands, pouring out of angry B cells that had traveled from her bloodstream to her brain.

MS usually arrives softly, a lamb, not a lion. Nagging numbness in a leg, a touch of blurred vision, or a dizzy spell. Explosions are unusual, but this is what befell Andrea. And for MS to begin with a change in behavior was even rarer. Young people with MS often recover from the first few episodes, but as attacks pile up over months and years, brain damage accumulates, recovery falters, and permanent disability takes hold. At the time, the outlook for most patients was a wheelchair by midlife, and for some, a helpless bedbound state. Andrea's prognosis was not even that good. She had a ferocious case, the likes of which I'd never seen.

She'd need to recover mostly on her own, healed by her body's natural capacity for repair, by her brain's resilience, but she would never regain her former level of function. There was little that we could do for her MS. No treatments existed then except for steroids, and these barely worked.

I returned to her bedside frequently that night, checking on her breathing, sitting by her side for a few minutes each time. ICU policies restricted visitors to short 15-minute stays during daytime hours only, but the nursing staff made an exception for Andrea, rolling in a reclining chair-bed so that one of her parents could be with her, speak to her, touch her shoulder, throughout the night. Sometimes rules are meant to be broken. Each time I checked in on Andrea, I'd also speak with her parents, comfort them as best I could, answer questions, and let them know what to expect in the coming days. Her mom's quiet sobbing and dad's look of total devastation remain etched in my memory.

Andrea seemed unable to understand anything that was said by that point, but I always assume that all patients, even those in deep coma, might comprehend more than we think, so what is said at the bedside should always be encouraging and never frightening. Young clinicians must be taught this simple but profoundly important rule, an axiom of the Hippocratic oath to "*first of all, do no harm.*"

The next morning, I met Dr. Fisher in the intensive care unit, and we stepped away to review my findings and plan the next steps. Andrea's mom brought me coffee and a donut.

"You've been up all night; you must be exhausted and hungry," she said.

I also met Andrea's boyfriend, her high school sweetheart

who'd just arrived from Virginia, a lanky and clean-cut young man who radiated goodwill and confidence that all would be well. Youth is courageous, but also clueless. Happily, though, his presence buoyed everyone's spirits.

But love and prayers would be no match for Andrea's illness. Faced with what would prove to be one of the most aggressive forms of MS, Andrea declined rapidly. Loss of speech and ability to swallow, cough, and breathe was followed by total paralysis on the right side of her body, and then weakness on the left. Simple tasks that we take for granted, like brushing our teeth or holding a book, were now impossible. She couldn't even sit unless strapped to a chair or bed. Within a few days, it became clear that surgery would be needed to create openings in her throat and stomach for insertion of permanent breathing and feeding tubes.

This was the saddest and most unfair thing I'd ever seen in medicine.

Medicine moved at a different pace in the 1970s. If someone was sick, they'd stay in a hospital for days, weeks, even months. They weren't "stabilized" then moved 72 hours later to some dark back room at a "post-acute" skilled nursing facility. And resident physicians knew nothing of today's work hour limits. We worked sometimes all night every other night, with 2 days off every 14 days. It was a brutal schedule, but it allowed time to connect with patients, to observe suffering at close hand, and to really understand what patients need from their physicians beyond a brisk checkup and diagnosis. Relationships were formed, and patients, their families, and caregivers could bond and get to know each other, often in the early hours of the morning.

I cared for Andrea for the next three weeks, long enough to see her level off and leave the intensive care unit for a large private room with a fireplace. I'd see her each day on morning and evening rounds, and sometimes, when things were quiet in the hospital, I'd come around just to say hello. I met her colleagues from work, her siblings, and her friends. So many people loved her and cared about her.

Her acute medical needs were now mostly behind her, and she'd soon be transferred for rehabilitation. She had made only marginal progress, though. She could now understand what was said to her, respond to simple yes/no questions by nodding or shaking her head, and even vocalize a few indistinct words when the tracheotomy tube was closed, but her terrible paralysis, complete on the right side and partial on the left, was unchanged. It would be a long road back, against long odds for recovery. I explained to her parents that now she needed time to see if her body was strong enough to heal, at least partially. They asked if I'd be willing to care for Andrea after she was discharged. Of course I would.

Several months passed before I saw Andrea again. It was a Sunday afternoon, and I was visiting her for a special occasion at the chronic care facility across from our hospital where she now lived. Entering the building's family room—a solarium—I saw her, seated in a wheelchair, strapped in place at the shoulders so that she wouldn't slump over, still paralyzed on the right side, breathing tube in place, but she was now able to speak more clearly, albeit haltingly, when the tracheotomy was closed. When she saw me, she smiled and whispered that she'd hoped that I would come. I bent over to give her a hug.

The high school sweetheart from Virginia, now her fiancé, stood to her left. They were getting married the next week and had organized a little party for us, her physicians and caregivers.

She was wearing a white gown; her hair was lovely, her makeup perfect. She looked beautiful and radiated happiness. Her folks were there, standing by her side. The sun sparkled through unwashed windows in the otherwise drab room, illuminating the faded green paint on the walls and old-fashioned vinyl chairs mostly used for sleeping by family members of countless patients, hoping against hope that their loved ones, stricken with one gruesome brain disease or another, might someday recover.

On this day, the bare, undecorated room was alive as never before, with flowers, balloons, and photos of the couple brought in for the occasion, enriched with friends who prepared food and passed out champagne—and soft drinks for us, the physicians on call. There was music, toasts, and hugs. It was the most beautiful bridal shower I'd ever seen.

And as I was leaving, her parents called out to me in the hallway.

"Please accept this gift. We are so grateful for all that you've done for our daughter, and for us. We hope that you will remember Andrea."

A small, blue Tiffany box, and inside a shimmering glass turtle paperweight. It still sits on my desk.

* * *

I decided right there that this common, crippling disease of young adults would be my life's work. MS robs people of basic functions that are usually taken for granted—vision, sensation, motor strength, coordination, bladder control, and sometimes, as with Andrea, even the ability to speak, eat, or breathe independently. Equally difficult is that MS imparts a sense of uncertainty, as lifelong as the disease. Questions abound. Will I have more attacks? Am I going to need a wheelchair? Should I abandon my career plans? What should I tell my loved ones? The future becomes clouded in doubt.

My inability to provide answers to these questions would drive and inspire me in the years to come.

Four decades later, I'd finally have some answers, some very good answers, and would stand on a podium before thousands of neurologists to unveil the results of a new treatment that would change the face of MS. This is the story of how it all happened.

CHAPTER 2

Provenance

Multiple sclerosis is a disease of the immune system and the brain. The immune system, designed to protect us against invading microbes, misidentifies nerve cells and their myelin coverings as foreign. This leads to an autoimmune attack—the body turning against itself. Normally, each nerve cell connects with thousands of others via electrical signals, but when myelin is attacked, the nerves short-circuit, like frayed power cords. Over time, the connections are lost, nerve cells die, and symptoms of brain disease appear.

These two subjects—troubles with the immune system and troubles with the brain—have been on my mind for as long as I can remember. I'm always trying to make connections between early events and my later choices in life, lining them up to create a coherent story. By linking events together, I can make better sense of the world and anticipate the future. However, I also know that these tales, built on cause-and-effect progressions, might deceive me as often as not. What does seem certain, however, is that random happenings, good and bad, played huge roles in how it all unfolded.

My own immune system has always been overactive. Asthma, allergies, and eczema have been my constant companions. Substances that are in no way dangerous—ragweed, mold, or dust—cause my immune system to inflame whatever portal they enter—lungs, throat, or skin. I was frequently ill with a vicious streak of the asthma that runs in the family. It was there when I was very young in New Orleans; was a constant presence throughout my youth in New York, disrupting sports and physical activities; and remained an irritant during college and early career years in Boston. And it always flared up in bucolic places, lakes and farms and woods.

Some of my earliest memories are of my mother spending time with me at my grandparents' home in New Orleans, under a bridge table covered by a sheet, a vaporizer spraying a fine mist so that I'd have healthier air, and then decamping to the beach to escape the harmful "pollen." She'd place cool water sponges over the itchy and painful patches of eczema on my skin, bloody from scratching in my sleep. Mom would keep lists of the many foods and medicines that would cause my lips to swell, throat to tighten up, or skin to erupt in a rash. Every leaf and blade of grass was poison ivy to my skin. And after we moved north to New York, there were years of expensive, and totally ineffective, weekly shots administered by well-meaning but clueless allergists, like the mustachioed Dr. Schnittke, who'd inject the potions into my arm as he chain-smoked in my face. The concoctions were adjusted each year based on my sensitivities to a panel of allergens injected under the skin of my back, a painful checkerboard of punctures that I repeatedly endured. He'd also use the results—against extracts of pollen, mold, hay, dander, and other things—to recommend where in the countryside my asthma would magically improve that summer. None of this worked on me, or on most anyone else. But because the doctor was always right, even though my symptoms only worsened in the dank lakeside cabins and funky motels, we never reconsidered the country cure theory.

In those days, clinical immunology was two parts alchemy, one part science.

In my eighth year, I was able to go to summer camp. I had no idea that Surprise Lake Camp in the Catskills was basically a social service organization for disadvantaged kids. It surrounded a magnificent lake—with a real diving board, just like in the movies—where I learned to swim. And the nights were the most amazing part of it all: there were so many stars. We'd never see stars like that in the city, and the sounds of the night—crickets, birds, and other critters, were unlike anything I'd ever heard.

But I couldn't breathe. The asthma inhalers that I carried with me and used several times every day worked well enough during daytime, but when evening came I'd be bent over, gasping for air, struggling for every breath. It would get even worse in the middle of the night. And each night Dave, the lead counselor, walked with me, or carried me, back to the main building, where a nurse clad in white was waiting. I needed medicine, quickly, and received shots, pills, and more inhalers. Dave would often stay up with me most of the night until finally I collapsed from exhaustion.

Despite my difficult nights, I loved the time at camp. I swam, played baseball and volleyball, and on rainy days made lanyard keychains for everyone in my family. One day, as a special treat, we were taken horseback riding to a cowboy campfire. Dave was with me all of the time, administering medications several times daily, checking to see that I could breathe reasonably well, and keeping me company during the long nights. When things were at their worst, he'd flash a crooked smile and tell me stories.

When the day came that my folks were to pick me up, we rode a bus to the gathering place. Dave and I rode together. When we reached the destination, I saw my folks and brother David out the window and hurried off to greet them. But then I remembered Dave and ran back onto the bus. Dave and I hugged for what seemed like the longest time, until I had to go. I never saw him again.

I'll never forget Dave's acts of kindness. I think of him each morning as I head to the hospital, remembering his humanity, and thanking him by acting in the same way toward my patients, as best I can.

In the future we will have computer programs that massively improve diagnosis and make treatment more democratic, efficient, effective, and accessible; prototypes for these already exist in clinics today. But physicians care for the soul as well as the body. So while what the computer does will far outstrip my knowledge, I'll always have skills that it lacks. No computer will be able to stare into a frightened patient's eyes, hold a hand, or touch a shoulder, even if the software can make the right decisions guided by encyclopedic medical data and detailed knowledge of each patient's biology, proclivities, and preferences. Embed the programs in human avatars that wear long white coats and resemble kindly Dr. Kildare, I'm still confident that computers will continue to work for physicians, not replace them.

This is because the caring part of medicine is as important as the science.

* * *

Troubles with the nervous system—neurology—was the other steady presence in my early life.

My brother Howard was born just a few weeks before my eighth birthday. Dad returned from the hospital and told us that Howard was sick and that he and Mom had to stay for a few days, which turned into a few weeks. Then followed news that my mother's parents, Grandma Rose and Grandpa Barney, were moving from New Orleans to New York to stay with my younger brother David and me, maybe permanently, but at least until Mom and Howard could come home. Dad picked them up at the train station. They brought presents—toys and clothes. Joy and excitement to see them after so many months apart!

Secure in the safety of home and family, with no experience of upheavals, it never crossed my mind that everything that I'd taken for granted was being turned upside down with one single stroke of ill fortune. It should have been obvious. I'd hear the adults whispering in the other room but paid it little mind, and I wouldn't even have known what to make of the information if it had been shared.

Howard had been born listless, barely moving, and with a dusky color, all signs of inadequate oxygen carried to the brain. He was fighting for his life. His physicians were uncertain if he'd make it. Only decades later did I learn that my frantic, frightened, tearful mom was so distraught that she'd been placed on 24-hour watch over concerns that she might hurt herself.

When Mom came back home, finally, while Howard was still in the hospital, she told us that nobody knew if he'd grow up normally, that we'd just have to wait, hope, and pray.

Our prayers were not enough. As Howard grew, the progress my parents hoped for never came: he'd never be able to walk, talk, or do much of anything on his own. It was a brain problem, Mom said, called mental retardation. Howard would laugh whenever I came into his room, and we'd play together, mostly rolling on the floor or watching TV. We became really good friends. After a while Mom would let me take him outside for walks in his stroller.

Children can be mean, especially when confronted with something that they don't understand. In fourth grade, someone started a rumor that we locked my brother up in the house, chained to a wall in the attic, kept him a prisoner. It's amazing that kids could believe this, but it escalated. Soon many of the boys were pointing fingers, laughing, saying nasty things like my brother was a monster, and excluding me from their lunch table.

One day I challenged the ringleader, a big kid, to a fight at 3 o'clock outside the school. Everyone was there, gathered in a circle around us. He put up his fists like a real boxer, and rat-a-tat-tat, within a few seconds, he gave me, as fighters say, a shoeshine. Mom nursed my black eye and bloody mouth, and when Dad heard about this, the boxing lessons began, though I didn't much take to them. I didn't need the lessons anyway; this was the only fight I'd ever have. The taunting soon stopped, and kids who used to tease would now sometimes even stop to chat when I was wheeling Howard around the neighborhood to the ice cream shop or the five-and-dime.

What had happened to my brother? Why was he so severely handicapped, mentally and physically? When she was still in the hospital, my mom was told by a nurse—or maybe it was an aide, she couldn't be sure—that he'd been "dropped," or might have been dropped, shortly after birth. A terrible fall might have explained a brain injury, but didn't account for another medical problem—abnormally high fevers. Whenever Howard was ill, his temperature would spike precipitously, sometimes above 107 degrees Fahrenheit. The doctors couldn't figure out why. I now know that it was pneumonia caused by aspiration of food and secretions down the windpipe and into his lungs, because the swallowing reflexes in my brother's brain were not working properly. Andrea had the same problem, but we could protect her lungs by inserting tubes for feeding and breathing. Without similar interventions, which never could have been monitored at home, Howard was sure to have episode after episode of severe aspiration and pneumonia. But in those days, the physicians blamed his fevers on a faulty immune system, said that he couldn't fight infections properly. In our neighborhood, doctors worked out of converted living rooms and opened books in front of patients to see what to do.

Howard's birth also gave rise to our family's great migration. My grandparents never returned to New Orleans, and Mom's brother Sandy and sister Rochelle soon followed their parents north to New York City. They were there when we needed them most, helping Mom care for her damaged baby, providing love and comfort to my brother and me.

Dad's parents pulled away. They told my folks that they worked hard all week and needed happiness on the weekends.

* * *

Our first home in New York was at Springfield Court, a complex of cookie-cutter garden apartments in Bayside Queens, where a tight-knit community of mostly young families lived, with many kids around my age. There were unlocked front doors with mats that said "Welcome" and meant it. The residents constantly convened on the shared porches, sitting on bridge chairs, drinking beer, talking, laughing, listening to transistor radios.

Mom's best friend Janet was the social anchor of the women's group, the event planner, the loudest talker and laugher. Compact, with short, bobbed hair, and full of life until one summer day when she collapsed during a late-night mahjong game—an epileptic seizure from a brain infection, we were told. She was near death for many days, husband at her side, the other moms pitching in to help with their two kids.

Janet survived, but she was away in rehab for what seemed like forever. I'd hear the moms talking on the porch.

"Her mind is shot," they'd say.

Slowly, over months, seasons changed and the conclaves on the porch gave way to school and cold weather. Families turned inward. The summer community, with its long evenings, warmth, and fireflies, was no more. The other moms stopped asking "How is she doing?" and moved on with their lives.

Then one day, without warning, I saw Janet. But she wasn't Janet anymore. Placid, smiling, exchanging only simple social pleasantries—"How are you?" "Beautiful day, isn't it?"—and behind the eyes no one was home. She had no idea who or where she was. On rare occasions we'd see her outside the apartment, limping along with her cane, but she'd mostly stay indoors. She was no longer a part of the mahjong group.

I'd learn only much later, in medical school, that Janet's demise was almost certainly caused by a virus that attacked the temporal lobes of her brain,* lasering in on the memory and personality parts, destroying the circuits that store our personal narratives and capacity to relate to others, empathize, read emotions, or assess the outside world in any meaningful way.

Janet no longer had anything to offer those around her.

* * *

In the third grade my best friend was a quiet, kind, and especially generous boy named Robert. He was unlike my other friends who were mostly noisy and pushy. He didn't even like sports. We'd go for walks, play games, and talk about books and TV shows. Once at his house we played a board game, the mystery game *Clue*. Beyond the game itself, I was especially taken with Robert's edition of the game, which was far more beautiful than ones I'd seen before. Robert noticed how much I liked it.

"I've played this game a lot and really don't need it anymore. Would you like to take it home? If we play it again you can bring it with you."

---

* Temporal lobe encephalitis is most often caused by infection with the herpes simplex virus. Herpes simplex is present in almost all healthy adults and is the cause of benign cold sores, but for reasons still obscure, it occasionally attacks the temporal lobes of the brain.

He was a wonderful friend.

One day I walked into the kitchen and heard Mom on the phone. Her back was turned to me, and the long curly cord of the wall-mounted phone was stretched so tightly that she was nearly out the back door and into the yard. She spoke in a hushed voice, a conversation clearly not meant for me to hear. But she mentioned Robert's name again and again, saying how sorry she was. A few minutes later, she sat me down.

"That was Robert's mom. Honey, Robert is very sick. He's in the hospital. He has a brain tumor and needs an operation to get better."

"Will he be OK?"

"The doctors don't know yet, but he won't be able to play for a while. Let's send a letter to let him know that we hope he'll be better soon. Maybe you could draw a picture of the *Clue* game and write that you'll play together as soon as he's back home."

I remember thinking that everything would be fine after my friend had his operation.

But Robert was gone for a very long time, and when he returned, our play dates moved to his apartment because he was no longer allowed to go outdoors. Then another long period where I didn't see him at all.

Many months later, Mom told me that Robert would come to play at our house but that this would probably be the last time we'd be able to play together.

We played in the backyard, went in the wading pool, had snacks, walked down the block. I had to move slowly, as he could no longer run or even walk very well. Mom said that I should hold on to his arm because he couldn't see clearly. We couldn't play *Clue* anymore, but still had fun. And at the end of the day his mom picked him up in front of our house. I remember waving goodbye, feeling bewildered.

I never saw Robert again. One day, several weeks later, Mom

told me that he had died. This was terribly sad, she said, even worse because his parents had no other children. She hugged me, wiped my tears away, and told me that I was lucky to have had such a good friend.

I had no idea what a brain tumor was or what it meant to have cancer. I didn't know that the cancer couldn't be removed because it wasn't solid, like a walnut. Instead, tiny flecks of cancer were budding up all over his brain, each then gradually spreading out, bit by bit, like crabgrass, until the normal parts of his brain were entirely overrun.

His parents had tried every medical intervention available. They knew that surgery wouldn't cure their son, but at least the terrible headaches might go away for a while. It was impossible to know if the chemotherapy did any good at all, and its side effects were terrible; the vomiting and weight loss were bad enough, but the drugs also made his eyes sensitive to sunlight so he couldn't even leave the house when the drugs were in his system. It must have seemed cruel to give him this poison, but they were desperate to give their beloved son every possible chance. And when so much of his brain tissue had been taken over that he couldn't play with his friends or experience joyful things, the treatment was stopped; it would no longer bring him any benefit.

How could a child understand any of this?

CHAPTER 3

Unconventional Roots

Years later, as a young neurology resident, I sat with my mentor, Charles Miller Fisher, in the autopsy suite at Massachusetts General Hospital, looking at the base of a brain that we'd just removed from a formaldehyde-filled bucket. At the bottom of our brains is a group of variably sized blood vessels that connect with each other, partially in some people and completely in others. Through these connections, blood flow can be redirected from one vessel to another when needed, improving perfusion to an injured ("ischemic") part of the brain and preventing a stroke. The great neuroanatomist Thomas Willis recognized in 1664 that these vessels form a "circle"—more of a hexagon, actually—and for the next 350 years the circle of Willis has been a central feature of human neuroanatomy taught to medical students everywhere.

"Stephen, if you were looking at this for the first time in the 1600s, would you have recognized these blood vessels as connected in a circle?" Fisher asked me.

"No, Dr. Fisher," I replied, "I don't think that I would have."

"Of course you would have!" he replied.

Seeing new relationships was not my forte. But curiosity and persistence, traits that I certainly did have, proved to be even more important qualities for a future medical scientist. I sometimes tell students that one difference between basic and clinical science is that the former places its highest value on creative leaps of thought—think Darwin or Einstein—and the latter on discoveries that improve people's lives. A clinician may make immensely important advances, figuring out the cause of disease and developing new lifesaving therapies through methods that might seem unoriginal or uncreative to the pure scientist. In clinical science, resilience and an ability to stay on course, despite storms and setbacks, often determines who reaches the finish line. And for those traits, I can thank my mom.

* * *

Many poor girls who grew up in the Deep South during the Great Depression enjoyed sports, but most were satisfied to be spectators or cheerleaders. Not my mom—she was always a participant. What drove her, at five feet and three inches tall, to become a pole vaulter? And what possessed her, as a high school senior, to park herself in the outer office of New Orleans mayor Robert Maestri for two full days until he'd see her?

"I need a scholarship to go to LSU! My momma and papa can't afford the fifty-dollar annual tuition," she pleaded. "And they always vote for you!"

The mayor was charmed.

"OK, li'l girl; heyah's a fou'-year scholarship, but remembuh to tell yo' folks to vote fuh Mayuh Maestri."

She did. And they did.

Louisiana State University changed Mom's life, not to mention the fortunes of the entire family. She earned room and board by lifeguarding at the LSU pool, even though she didn't know how to swim, and by tutoring football players—famous ones like Y. A. Tittle, Alvin Dark,* and Steve Van Buren. Some

---

* Alvin Dark was best known for football at LSU, but would later become even more famous as an all-star professional baseball player and manager.

were illiterate, and her job was to somehow get them through the semester, which she did.

When the four years came to an end, Mom went back to the mayor's office and asked if he could cross out her name on the scholarship certificate and write in the name of her baby brother Sandy. Sandy had barely made it through high school, but Maestri was accommodating.

"Of course, li'l girl; but remembuh now you tell yo' mammy and daddy to vote fuh Mayuh Maestri."

New Orleans is a colorful town, and Maestri was a quintessential New Orleans politician. He rose to power as an acolyte of Huey Long and quickly became known for his neighborhood outreach and open-door policies. Any citizen could just walk in, but even more important, could share in the patronage.* And with her soft Southern drawl and sweet disposition, even as a teenager Mom could play the system like a Stradivarius.

Mom didn't know or care that there were boundaries for poor girls in the South of the 1930s. In high school, she tried to join the FBI, but when a federal agent arrived at the house unannounced for a background check, her parents thought he'd come to deport them back to Poland. Mom's career as a sleuth was over, but she was soon hired as an assistant to Charles E. Fenner Jr. of the New Orleans firm Fenner & Beane. They were a Southern commodities company, and Mom's job was to count cotton bushels. Through merger, the company would soon be renamed Merrill Lynch, Pierce, Fenner & Beane. In later years Mom would get advanced degrees in education at night school, dedicate her life to the education of disabled kids, become a decorated long-distance runner, and care for her clan

---

* Maestri had struck a deal with the mobster Frank Costello. New Orleans would overlook existing laws against gambling and prostitution and in return get a cut of the action.

like an overly protective grizzly bear. At age 90, she was still secretary of her bike club.

* * *

I learned to be curious and unhurried from Mom's brother, my Uncle Sandy. Compact, strong, and gregarious, Uncle Sandy was also an amateur boxer and a collector of exotic friends and experiences. And above all, a gifted talker. Sandy needed a guide to get across the street lest he stop to engage with each stranger he'd pass. He'd draw them out and relate to them, whether they were corner shoeshine guys, athletes, or celebrities.

It was pretty much impossible not to like Sandy.

Each summer, my dad would go off for three weeks of military training, and Sandy, also a reservist but still a bachelor then, would swoop us away on a vacation tour. The planning was minimal, the pace slow, and we often had no idea where we'd be the next day. We wouldn't miss a single historical marker, log cabin, natural bridge, glass-bottom boat, or cave. Every Abe Lincoln birthplace had to be seen,* and at each site the life stories of caretakers, gardeners, and tour guides revealed.

Seven of us would pile into Sandy's white Chevy Impala, three in the front and four in the rear. My brother David and me, Mom, her parents, Mom's younger sister Rochelle, and, behind the wheel, Sandy. We'd often sleep in the car, sometimes in a parking lot behind a Howard Johnson's where the bathroom facilities were far superior to those at most roadside rest stops. But some evenings we'd search for a motel.

---

* Fragments of the original one-room log cabin in Sinking Spring, Kentucky, where Lincoln was reportedly born, were dismantled and rebuilt for display in different places. Some planks were repurposed for a newer home nearby, and others used to build the facsimile now on display at the Abraham Lincoln Birthplace National Historical Park.

Here's how it was done. First, we'd wait until it was late, sometimes after midnight. We'd cruise down the motel strip of each small Southern town, choosing ones that seemed affordable, had signs that said "VACANCY," and were likely to soon close down for the night. We'd drive up to the entrance, and Mom and Sandy would go into the small office, leaving the rest of us waiting in the car, sometimes for a very long time.

They'd ring the desk bell and the owner would appear, usually emerging from a small apartment behind the office wall. They'd speak for a few minutes and then walk outside together, the manager dangling the room keys to show the accommodations. And then the haggling would begin.

We'd watch the progress from our car, rolling down the windows to listen in, my brother and I desperately praying that they'd be successful, mostly so we could cool off in the fabulous swimming pool on the front lawn. The negotiations could get intense. Always two rooms, one for each gender, and secured only after multiple failed attempts, with the bargaining sometimes ending in shouts and threats by the innkeeper to call the police. Our price point was 12 dollars, 6 dollars per room, a sum that usually, but not always, would work in the rural South in the 1950s. Sixty years later, we still recite to each other a few of the greatest hits, like this one from Gatlinburg, Tennessee.

"Goddamn it, Jesus Christ, fo' chrissakes, hell no! Ah did everything ah could. Ah gave ya extra towels an' a room with one of the air coolers, but that's it. I git fifteen dollars a room and ah'm givin' you two for fourteen. But ah ain't gon' down to twelve. Now git the hell out of here, fa God sakes!"

Mom and Sandy would then go outside, not back in the car but just outside the office, and after five minutes or so they'd walk back in and start bidding again. Of course, even rooms that supposedly went for 15 dollars a night often weren't perfect—this was before the era when national chains brought some level of consistency to motels. The rooms sometimes had so many spiders, beetles, or wall-mounted creatures (and on one occasion flying bats), that the car seemed preferable. But the car did not have the swimming pool, or a black-and-white Philco television with rabbit ears. I also remember how respectfully my family, and especially Grandma, treated the rooms once we secured them. In the morning, before departure, she'd thoroughly scrub each room and make the beds—"so that the owner would know we're a clean family"—and leave two dollars by the pillow in each room for housekeeping. Then, she'd go back to the front office to say goodbye, and sometimes exchange addresses. Southern manners.

* * *

Sandy, who was blessed with a golden voice, also expanded my horizons. After the Korean War, he returned home a hero and soon landed jobs announcing local prizefights. He parlayed the contacts he'd made while an amateur boxer, persistence, and his magnetic personality to higher rungs in the world of play-by-play, and soon was broadcasting professional boxing.

This was my introduction to an exotic new world filled with braggadocio, courage, and pain. I was hooked. I met every boxer or sports icon imaginable. Jack Dempsey came to our house for dinner and a walk through the neighborhood. Another time, a 17-year-old kid named Cassius Clay, just out of the Olympics, talked up a storm on a Manhattan street, made up poetry, and predicted great things. I saw Sugar Ray Robinson at the twilight of his career; hung out at Jake LaMotta's favorite watering hole; and watched Satchel Paige, maybe pushing 60, pitch for the Indians.

Everything was going smoothly until Sandy made a fateful error, broadcast live to the world, when he mistakenly introduced a drunk who'd stumbled into the ring as Heavyweight Champion Michael Spinks. An understandable faux pas, scores of people were popping in and out of the ring during prefight introductions, to shake hands with the combatants, to wish them well. Embarrassing for sure, but not deserving of the death sentence that followed: Sandy was banished from boxing, at least for a time. And while in exile, he pivoted to the wrestling ring, where the world was even more colorful and the narratives much more engaging to an impressionable youngster from the dreary outreaches of Queens.

Boxers were interesting, sure, but they couldn't hold a candle to the wrestlers, not to Killer Kowalski and the other supercharged characters. Backstage I'd watch the stars getting ready for their "grudge" matches, baby-faced good guys, outfitted as superheroes or all-American surfers, yukking it up with the heels—untamed jungle wild men, malevolent sheiks, peroxide-coiffed villains—laughing, playing cards, sharing stories and beer before the match. And afterward, they'd nurse their injuries, repair the chairs clobbered over heads, pack up the outfits, and leave for the next roadshow.

It was better by far to be a heel. The bad guys had more creative acts, and it was fun to taunt the fans.

On one trip together we ate at the Pickrick in Atlanta, a fried chicken shack owned by former Georgia governor Lester Maddox. The old racist still hung out at the lunch counter. One dark night on a quiet country road in rural Louisiana we stumbled upon a Ku Klux Klan rally complete with scores of hooded, white-robed crusaders, a huge cross burning, all in full view of our family, transfixed by the scene despite knowing that as Jews we could be their next target.

Sandy's sleeping habits added to his legend. He slept 90 minutes each night. That's all he needed. He'd spend most of the night reading papers, *Ring* and other boxing magazines, wrestling ones too. Usually in the bathroom so he wouldn't disturb his wife. Until 3 a.m. Then he'd sleep some, but was up at 4:30 for the long commute from Brooklyn to the Long Island school where he taught history, leaving plenty of time before 8 a.m. class. Energy radiating out of his eyeballs.

"Never tired," he'd always say.

* * *

I've always enjoyed getting to know my patients as people, gradually and over time, meeting their families, sharing their joys, and helping with their sorrows. I've been ministering to some for nearly a half century. It's one of the great pleasures of medicine, equal to the satisfaction of caring for the physical ailments. It's easy for me to relate to people who are different or eccentric, a consequence, I think, of my colorful childhood.

CHAPTER 4

The Young Scholar

In New Orleans, we lived in my grandparents' apartment on the second floor of a ramshackle two-family wooden home. My first school was just down the block from our house.

One day in kindergarten I realized that I could read. I don't think that I was specifically taught by anyone; it just seemed to come naturally. The teacher gave me a few books to take home and I recall running up the back steps, declaring loudly that I knew how to read books. Mom didn't believe me, but we sat down with my grandmother and I rattled off the words of the early reader, page by page. They declared me a prodigy, a mixed blessing when in future years I repeatedly fell short of their expectations.

I was also lefthanded, as lefty as a lefty could possibly be. My grandparents hated it, as did my teachers. Not to worry, my first-grade teacher said, because with my grandfather's help, this could be corrected before the end of the year. They tied my left arm to my chest with a belt to force me to use my right hand, making sure that it remained in place both at school and at home. But it didn't work, because I couldn't do it. Try as I might, I just could not write legibly. Finally, they gave up. At school, another unrepentant lefty and I were assigned permanent seats in the back row on the left side of the classroom so that our elbows wouldn't bother the other students.

I didn't notice that there were no Black students anywhere in the school, even though New Orleans was 70 percent African American. It was the 1950s and schools were segregated.*

Summers in New Orleans were especially hot. No air conditioning, but there was always Pontchartrain Beach. We'd go in the evening; it was too hot during the day. The lake water was tepid, brownish, brackish, and silty, and in addition to the undertow, we had to keep an eye out for horseshoe crabs, snapping turtles, and the occasional wandering alligator. But still it was a great place, with swimming pools, carnival rides and booths, memorable fries served in a paper cone, hot buttered corn, and gator pies.

* * *

After we moved to New York, my fast start as an academic quickly sputtered. There was no simple explanation, but in part it was too many distractions: sports, sci-fi and detective stories, late-night TV movie marathons, a busy paper route and greeting card business, too much daydreaming, topped off by a general lack of interest in school. Third grade went particularly poorly.

Mrs. Rosen's class was like one of those soap operas my mother's friends would watch, but with even more drama. Once during a current events discussion, I parroted something my father told me, that the Arabs deserved a home in Israel. She turned to me, welling up with tears, gesticulating wildly.

"You don't know what you're saying! This is Israel's land! Don't you know that the Nazis ripped out the ovaries of Jews?"

She did some sort of pantomime to illustrate the point.

"How would you feel if they ripped out your ovaries?"

---

* A hotel in our neighborhood had a sign in the front window that said "No Negroes or Jews Allowed."

I was eight years old and had no idea what she was talking about.

* * *

In the spring, my parents were summoned to school for a group meeting with Mrs. Rosen, the principal, the guidance counselor, and the social worker. Everyone but the child welfare officer was there.

"There's no question that your son is capable," began Mrs. Rosen. "But his grades are terrible. We can't figure out why he is doing so poorly, and thought you could help us understand. Is there something going on at home that we should be aware of?"

"Everything is fine," Mom replied. "I have no idea why he isn't doing better."

"Has his behavior changed? Does he seem depressed?"

"No, he seems perfectly happy."

My folks spoke to me about the meeting after dinner that night in my bedroom, without my brother David around. Unusual, because we never had secret discussions. Dad said that the teachers' union was run by communists, but I should still try harder in class. I promised I would.

* * *

Small differences in age seem so important to most kids, but not to my brother David and me. We were two and a half years apart, separated in school by three classroom grades. In those early days, when family and home were the center of life, we were a team. We did everything together, slept in the same room, wore identical clothes, played streetball with the same friends, took evening baths together. We'd walk to school holding hands. He was my younger brother, and my job was to protect him. But we were both slowly growing up, and our worlds were enlarging, perspectives changing. Neither of us could pinpoint exactly when this first happened. It came on so gradually, over months, over years. It might have started when I turned 10, maybe 11. Maybe in fourth grade. Our proclivities, interests, personalities diverged. We were becoming different people, and we were no longer a team.

David was more handsome, athletic, and well-liked than me. Soon he'd hang out with the cool kids, play drums and sing in a rock band that actually got gigs. Real gigs. He'd have girlfriends, lots of them, win popularity contests, get elected to things. He was a BMOC (Big Man On Campus), while it was already clear that I was more of a wonk. My few friends were mostly like me. We all thought we'd be successful. But I was still a slacker, not turning my aspirations into anything approaching a sustained academic effort.

* * *

I mostly sleepwalked through the next few years of school, deposited in what was referred to as "the dumb class," with the kids headed to vocational occupations, far away from my former classmates in the academic crowd.

My fourth-grade teacher was Mrs. Breen, a tall, stern brunette who wore tight-fitting clothes and a push-up bra. She seemed old to us, but was probably 35 at most. She'd disappear for hours at a time, down to the electrical room in the basement, where it was common knowledge that she was smoking cigarettes and carrying on with the maintenance man. We were left unsupervised, assigned to a "reading period" or told to watch a movie that she'd start on a large projector before scurrying off. So we'd mostly fend for ourselves.

Some days she'd bring her beau upstairs to witness little games that she choreographed, using the class as a prop. She taught us that pandemonium meant silence, and whenever she said, "Class, now let's have some pandemonium," we were to sit straight up in our chairs, hands clasped, lips pursed, no movement, perfectly silent. We obeyed, time and again, and each time the lovers would walk out of the classroom, hand in hand, howling with laughter.

Nothing beats a tip-top public education.

* * *

When you hit rock bottom, the only place to go is up. I didn't want to be grouped with the slow kids any longer. I was ready to rev up my effort, not wholeheartedly but modestly, gradually, incrementally. And by sixth grade, approaching my final turn in elementary school, I'd done well enough to vault into the number-one pole position, the elite class taught with great seriousness, though I was bottom half there, still a laggard, not reliably reading the assigned homework materials.

CHAPTER 5

Special Skills

My brother Howard was now three years old. He'd learned to crawl, but would never stand or walk independently. He'd laugh and babble but couldn't speak or understand words. He usually seemed happy as long as he wasn't hungry or sick, but sometimes, if not watched, he would bang his head against the wall. My brother loved whenever David or I came into his room; he'd greet us with a big smile and a joyful honking sound. We'd tickle him, roll over together, and play. Sometimes I'd pick him up, chest high, and carry him off to my bedroom, showing him my toys and playing on the bed together.

Mom set out to become an expert in childhood disabilities. She quickly became licensed to teach special education in the New York City public school system. Severely disabled youngsters just like my brother. It was a full-time job, nine to three each day, and as a Southern-style homemaker, she'd still do all of the cooking and cleaning.

Next, Mom decided that she needed a master's degree to understand the field in depth.

The best option was a program at Yeshiva University, located at a new Manhattan branch of the school on 57th Street and 5th Avenue, an easy ride on the F line. Two nights each week, after working all day and returning home to prepare dinner for Dad, leaving Howard with Grandma Rose or Beulah, an

African American housekeeper who lived nearby and helped with his care, Mom would bundle up David and me, and we'd travel by bus and subway to Manhattan. When we reached the school, we'd stop in the lobby on the first floor, where there was a fabulous Horn and Hardart automat where we could put nickels in the vending machines to get heavenly Salisbury steak (basically a hamburger minus the bun, drenched in brown gravy) and mashed potatoes, and apple pie for dessert. We'd then go upstairs with Mom and wait outside the classroom, playing or doing our homework while she was in class, then get back on the subway and return home.

Heavy, thick textbooks on subjects like early childhood education, childhood psychology, and special ed were stacked on Mom's bedstand and scattered on her bed. Pen and paper in hand, she'd take notes, study, and memorize late into the night. This went on for years, until she passed all the tests, almost satisfactorily. She needed a B average to get the degree, and was on track until she received a D in one course during the final semester. So, Mom went to the professor's office and told him that a D would not do; she needed a C to bring her average up to a B.

"I have to have a C in your course. What would it take get my grade changed?"

"It would take two fins," he replied—New York lingo for ten dollars.

No problem.

So, Mom got her master's degree, and on graduation day the whole family was there to share in the joy. She spent the next quarter century working with children just like Howard, and, as importantly, helping their moms, who blamed themselves just as she had. On many days she'd bring one or two of her kids home after school, kids from all backgrounds and ethnicities, and play with them and diaper and feed them until one of their parents could come home from work to pick them up.

* * *

Ryan Junior High School is where I learned how to pick locks. My friend Eddie Wagner taught me. Confident, always dressed in black, with a long ducktail greased to a slinky shine, Eddie was the coolest kid I knew. I'm not sure if he ever went to class. He lived in a walkup apartment with his mom, who'd sit in the living room glued to the TV, even in the middle of the afternoon, and his alluring, much older sister, all mascara and beehive hair piled high. She looked like a Ronette. His dad had disappeared long ago. I'd never tell my parents when I went there.

Eddie had outstanding powers of concentration and, as it turned out, was also an excellent teacher.

Each kid at school had a metal locker secured with a combination lock that opened with a three-digit code, first by turning clockwise, then counterclockwise but two full revolutions, then clockwise again to the third and final number. Eddie began at my locker, pressing his ear close to the lock as he slowly turned the dial. He had it in less than ten seconds. The key, he showed me, was to make very slow rotations while carefully listening to each click, like a roulette wheel. When the correct number hits, there is a subtle change to the tone of the click and a looser feel on the dial. Almost anyone can become a successful lock picker with proper training, practice, and attention to detail. In addition to its obvious benefit, it's also a good way to train the mind to concentrate.

Soon I had mastered the technique, and occasionally I would surprise friends—and years later my kids—by opening a lock whose combination had been forgotten. Like riding a bicycle, it's a skill that once acquired is never lost.

Eddie was cool, but he was also a bona fide juvenile delinquent and headed for big trouble. And over time it became clear that our friendship couldn't last. We went our separate ways.

CHAPTER 6

Hauser's Shoes

Dad's family were alphas—New Yorkers, fifth-generation German Jews, hard-boiled, thick-skinned, and successful. Dad's dad, Louis Hauser, was the original tough guy. Lou rescued his brother Mo from Europe at the dawn of World War II, brought him into his home, taught him English, and set him up as a salesman in his store on Liberty Avenue in Brooklyn: Hauser's Shoes. But as soon as Mo mastered the basics of the business, he opened a competing shoe store just across the street, even trying to hire away Grandpa Lou's best salesmen. Grandpa crushed him like a bug. I don't think they ever spoke again. Loyalty mattered to Grandpa, and as a young child I learned never to cross Dad's side of the family.

My dad had worked at Grandpa Lou's shoe store as a teenager. But Dad was a man of action, and everyone knew that there was no way he could be contained there. Sometime around 1942, at the age of 17, he quit and became a collegiate nomad, starting in the north and moving progressively southward, rapid fire from one college to another, like a slinky down a flight of stairs. When Georgia Tech didn't work out, he moved on to Louisiana State in Baton Rouge. There, he met Mom at a freshman dance, and that first night asked her to go steady. Grandma wouldn't allow it, but it was love at first sight for both Mom and Dad.

Dad had little interest in academics. He yearned to get into the war before it ended, and in June 1943 he turned 18 and enlisted. He became an Army paratrooper in the 503rd Regiment and was wounded in combat in a terribly bloody but ultimately successful jump on Fortress Corregidor in the Philippines.* When the war ended, he left his pet monkey in New Guinea, returned to New Orleans, and married Mom.

Dad was kind and caring, but could also be hot-headed. Once, when a driver cut him off, he jumped out of the car, ignoring Mom's pleas, and rolled up his sleeves to settle the score. On another occasion he started a fistfight in a futile attempt to desegregate a public bus in New Orleans. Years later, the neighborhood kids would refer to him as the Commandant, always in whispers. A few of my friends were afraid to come to our house. My dad was not someone you'd want to tangle with.

In the early 1950s, he tried to join the new astronaut program but was too tall to fit into the snug Mercury capsule, so he needed to find another calling.

Dad was always an artist, with musical and literary gifts, but foremost he was a visual genius. He could draw from memory, capturing the nuances of any scene precisely, the shadows, the detail. Boy, could he draw. And he instinctively knew how just a subtle tweak, in composition or palette, could transform a visual experience, make the landscape more magnificent, the face more expressive, the shoe more desirable. In fact, he'd soon launch his own women's shoe company based in Florence, Italy, receive accolades for his designs, then ascend the corporate ladder to ultimately lead the largest shoe company in

---

* On February 16, 1945, the 503rd Parachute Infantry Regiment, known as "the Rock Regiment," suffered more than 700 casualties in capturing the island held by more than 6,500 Japanese troops. A small drop zone was responsible for many fatalities; paratroopers were unintentionally dropped directly over their adversaries, some were killed crashing into each other during the drop, and strong winds blew others off course and over cliffs.

the United States, US Shoe Corporation, based in Cincinnati, Ohio. His friends included glamorous fashion designers, multilingual European businessmen, soldiers of fortune, and even a former Third Reich paratrooper, all of whom became part of our family's circle. And Dad remained an Army reservist for more than 20 years, teaching parachuting and martial arts to a generation of recruits.

I looked up to him with awe. His chiseled physique, dignified bearing, how he'd speak with just a few carefully chosen words. I knew I'd never match his courage or style, but from early childhood would hear that I was a chip off the old block. For starters, we looked alike, which helped a lot. On weekends I'd often wear the army uniforms he'd bring to me from the commissary, complete with backpacks and canteens and hats, field jackets festooned with rows of medals, mixtures of Dad's extras and my cub scout ones. Even in the hot humid summers. I was channeling Dad; I wanted to be like him.

Dad's accomplishments and the circles in which he walked were sources of pride for our entire family. Even tough Grandpa Lou was proud. Adding to the aura was the knowledge that success happened on Dad's own terms, even though the seeds were planted early in life, in that little shoe store that he hated on Atlantic Avenue in Brooklyn.

* * *

Unlike my dad, I loved everything about Hauser's Shoes.

In fact, I loved all sorts of work, it was in my blood. From age seven or eight I ran newspaper routes for the *Long Island Press*, sold cards and stationery for the Cheerful Card Company, secured contracts from neighbors to shovel their driveways after each snowfall, all providing cash in hand for the things I needed to buy: science fiction books of all kinds, comics, a TV for my room, and a transistor radio that could pick up Yankee games from almost anywhere, even the mountains. I bought science and magic kits, an ant farm, plastic soldiers and forts and Lionel trains, and had money left over to buy lavish birthday and anniversary gifts for my family.

And when I turned 12, I was finally allowed to work in the family shoe store, every Saturday, every holiday, sometimes even on Sundays when we needed to take inventory, or restock, or decorate the windows for the upcoming season.

My grandfather would pick me up early in the morning, and we'd drive to Brooklyn. It was more than a half-hour drive each way. Time for stories about his life, his friends, and what it was like when my dad was growing up just around the corner from the Liberty Avenue store. I learned that our roots were in Austria-Hungary, in present-day Ukraine, and that my ancestors had been farmers and ranchers on one side and brewers on the other. Beginning in the mid-19th century they scattered, some to the United States and later others to Palestine. I had no idea that my grandfather had been born in Austria and came to the United States as a six-year-old child. These were not the sorts of things that we ever spoke about at home.

Hauser's Shoes catered to children, women, and men alike. The age of specialization had not yet arrived. We were in the poorest part of town but stocked the fanciest brands: Wright Arch Preserver and Florsheim for men, Red Cross and US Shoe for women, Stride Rite for the kids. One-stop shopping—you could get special shoes for Sunday church, L. B. Evans slippers, and hi-top Converse Chuck Taylor All Star sneakers.

Jerry, an Eastern European Jew who Grandpa Lou had brought to the US to escape the Nazis, was Hauser's best salesman. Short and wiry, with a huge smile and crooked yellow teeth, a pencil lodged behind his ear to update the little notepad in his chest pocket that kept track of the "stock," Jerry was a genius at moving shoes that had been in the store for a decade, often in dusty, crushed boxes—think yellow pumps with a pink plastic flower on the toe. If the shoe didn't fit quite right, Jerry would take the pair to a hidden repair station behind the back wall near the small peep hole by Grandpa's desk and stretch out the spot that was too tight or add layers of pads to the toes and heels until the shoe was snug as a bug.

Jerry taught me the shoe business, starting with how to stack the shoes correctly on the shelves in the main room where they covered all four walls, floor to ceiling. I learned to check inventories, and then, during the busy Christmas season, I'd get to work with the customers, measuring shoe sizes with the wooden Ritz shoe sizer, and helping them try on the shoes using a stainless steel Florsheim shoehorn.

Jerry would check the fit by pressing against the toe up front and arch side to side. If the C width was a bit too wide, he'd say, "Try the Benny," lingo for B, a narrower shoe. And when I made the sale, the best part was blowing up a Hauser's Shoe Store balloon for the kids with the helium tank behind the cash register.

When I turned 13, Grandpa began to entrust me with the most important part of the business. Each Saturday afternoon at 4:30, when the store was settling down, all of the day's cash, sometimes more than $2,000, would be carefully rolled up into a ball secured with rubber bands. Grandpa would stuff it into my pocket with a deposit slip, and I'd quickly walk the two blocks down Liberty Avenue, passing by the ice cream parlor and candy store, to get to the bank before closing time at 5:00 p.m.

It was fortunate that Jerry and Grandpa trained me so well, because two years later, Jerry died suddenly, a heart attack they said, leaving the shoe store without a lead salesman. Grandpa mostly filled the gap, but I also helped by working extra shifts when needed. Grandpa supported Jerry's family for a very long time, but their hope that Jerry would someday be his successor was not to be.

CHAPTER 7

Jamaica High

Jamaica High is where I finally grew up. It was my first school that wasn't within walking distance of the house. I'd meet up with neighborhood friends, and together we'd take the city bus, quickly exiting our middle-class neighborhood, where each block was a perfect rectangle laid out with cookie-cutter houses on postage stamp parcels, then cross Union Turnpike into the impossibly opulent Jamaica Estates. There, the streets were no longer a grid but curved, with high fences, lush foliage, and houses mostly hidden except for the occasional turret or porch, a peek at the splendors within. When we neared Hillside Avenue, gateway to South Jamaica, the scene suddenly changed again, with ramshackle houses and graffiti.

Our school was integrated, but not really. While white and Black kids both went to school there, they lived in different neighborhoods, sat in different parts of the bus, and for the most part took different classes.

When we exited the bus, we'd pass through the gates of the school's thick iron fence, climb the stone stairs surrounded by majestic lawns, and ascend to the building itself. There were six huge wooden doors beneath the grand ionic columns. Once inside the front door it was white right, Black left. I'd turn right into a small, self-contained area reserved for high-achieving students (somehow, I was now part of this group). This was where I lived at Jamaica High.

The kids who turned left disappeared to parts unknown in the bowels of the school. I had no idea what went on there. The school was as segregated as anything I'd experienced in New Orleans. I'd see Black students in three places: on the bus, standing and talking on the steps of the school, and on the sports fields. Only rarely in the classroom.

Basketball was king, and though I loved the sport, I didn't have a chance. The team was impossibly talented. And tall, which I was not. So, I joined the track team, a haven for kids like me who liked team sports but weren't stars.

Our coach was Larry Ellis, who'd soon go on to fame when one of his students, Bob Beamon, a long jumper, went on to annihilate the world record by nearly two feet at the 1968 Mexico City Olympics. For the coach, Beamon's feat was a ticket out of Jamaica High, to Princeton University. And Beamon became a household word, an adjective, "beamonesque," signifying astounding athletic accomplishment. Beamon, who was Black, was a once-in-a-century track prodigy, but at Jamaica High even he focused on basketball.

Years later, describing his time at Jamaica High, Beamon said, "My high school was a jungle. You had to be constantly alert—ready to fight or run. If you joined one of the gangs, you might escape harm but you also might be in trouble the rest of your life. If you stayed decent, you stood a good chance of being clobbered every day. So I went hot and heavy for basketball—and I feel it saved me from being cut up. Basketball is big stuff in New York. If you're good in it, everybody respects you. Nobody would want to ruin your shooting eye or your shooting arm."*

---

* "Beamon Made Sport's Greatest Leap" by Larry Schwartz. Special to ESPN.com. (https://www.espn.com/sportscentury/features/00014092.html)

His description of Jamaica High is so different from mine as to be unrecognizable.

For the kids like me, Jamaica High was in its heyday, a pantheon of academic excellence. This was decades before it tumbled from "the best secondary school in the country" to a new designation as a "persistently dangerous school" that finally closed in 2014 due to longstanding failures in safety and performance. But this was a half century earlier, and Jamaica High was still the pride of Queens. And fate was on my side when I was placed in Louis Sparago's metallurgy class. He'd become a teacher as a last act after a long career in industry, he'd tell us, a chance to give back, satisfy an itch, and do something rewarding. He wasn't shy about sharing his opinion of the other science teachers at Jamaica High.

"They have no useful skills," he'd say, an impish smile beneath thick black glasses framing his bald head. "Back during the teachers' strike they had to sell encyclopedias. Nobody would hire them. Science has to be practical, otherwise it's just a mind game. I'm going to teach you useful stuff."

Parental consents in hand, every Thursday evening he'd take us to the Brooklyn Polytechnic Institute where we'd each be paired with a graduate student to assist with a thesis project and decipher a problem in metallurgy. We learned about elements, alloys, lattice structure, crystal growth. Amazing that trig and calculus were actually needed to get answers! I was assigned to a frumpy, bearded student whose shirt tail was usually hanging out on one side, the other stuffed into underwear peering over his beltline. To me he was Thomas Edison. His project was to develop ways to increase the strength and durability of steel. We prepared different alloys; tested various heating protocols; measured resilience, flexibility, and fatigue; and even used an electron microscope to observe our creations firsthand at astonishingly high resolution. And during these sessions and the long subway rides back and forth to Brooklyn each week, Mr. Sparago would encourage each of us. Not in a pushy way but enough to know that he believed in our potential. The Thursday night excursions continued for the entire school year, and not one of the dozen or so kids who signed up ever dropped out.

Practical science was something I could get into.

CHAPTER 8

Tragedy and Rebound

I was on my way out the door, headed to school, when the phone rang. A voice on the other end said, "Hello. Can I speak to your parents? I'm calling about Howard. This is very important."

It was April 30, 1965, 7:30 a.m. I'd known the moment the phone rang, knew even before I began to lift the handle on the purple, wall-mounted kitchen phone. I knew for certain that my brother Howard had died. Nobody ever called this early in the day, and I knew that there were ongoing concerns about my brother's health. For several months he'd been ill, off and on, with those mysterious sky-high fevers.

Dad, an early riser, had already left for work, and Mom was, as usual, rushing to get my brother and me out on time, making sure that we remembered our lunches in the fridge she'd prepared the night before. The moment we were out the door she'd be headed to PS 173, my former grade school, where she now worked as a teacher, helping severely handicapped children like my youngest brother. On this morning, Mom was wearing my favorite outfit, topped with a multicolored scarf that I thought made her look incredibly beautiful. More than 50 years later, I remember each detail, crystal clear, in slow motion.

I handed her the phone. She listened for a second, and

then screamed "*No!*" A gut-wrenching sound from the center of a wounded soul. She ran out, leaving the front door wide open, shouting, "I've got to find your father." Dad was long gone, though, and while it seemed like forever before she returned, it was probably no longer than five minutes. And by this time several neighbors were also in the house, trying to help however they could.

It had been about six months since Howard left the little room next to mine. My parents had intended to care for my brother at home, certainly while he was a child and later for as long as they could, but their plans collided with reality. By age seven, Howard had become too large to easily lift out of the reinforced crib and into the specially made stroller and too difficult to feed, change, and bathe. Increasingly unable to care for him properly and faced with the difficulty of finding the next in a steady stream of care attendants, my folks made the heartbreaking decision to move him to a facility dedicated to the care of severely disabled people.

We'd visit every weekend. It was far away in distant Westchester, my first time on the Taconic Parkway. The whole area was so much more beautiful than Queens. The towns resembled the pristine New England villages of my imagination, with village greens and steeples. A Jewish organization had taken over a majestic old building surrounded by fabulous lawns, and this was Howard's new home.

And there we'd spend afternoons in the sunshine with a picnic basket that my mom would fill with our favorite things—sandwiches, cookies, and homemade lemonade. I'd bring a book, usually science fiction or the Hardy Boys, plus the ever-present transistor radio tuned to baseball games. My brother always seemed fine, happy to see us and perfectly healthy, rolling over on the blanket, eating spoonfuls of vanilla ice cream that I fed him in the bright afternoon sun, and laughing as we played puppet games.

I took charge of the household that awful day, locating my dad and helping Mom when she returned. I recall almost nothing else from the days that followed my brother's death.

But one painful recollection from this period remains. I was spending the weekend at my grandparents' fancy apartment in Forest Hills, and my parents and David were soon to arrive for a special Sunday brunch of fresh bagels and lox. I'd gone shopping with my grandfather, who made sure that the bagels were well done and still warm and that the lox was the less salty "Nova Scotia" type. I was now in the kitchen with Grandma Essie, my Dad's mom, who was preparing the feast. We were chatting about something or other when she abruptly changed the topic.

"You shouldn't be sad," she told me. "It's a good thing that Howard died."

I don't think I said anything. I was surprised, but don't recall feeling angry or thinking much of anything except that my grandmother was wrong. While I later understood what she meant, I never figured out how she could say such a thing to me. He was my brother.

* * *

My mom never fully recovered from the guilt of having brought a handicapped baby into the world and then sending him away for custodial care where he would die far from home, alone, without anyone who loved him. She kept no pictures of Howard, it was just too heartbreaking to see them again, but the mental images couldn't be erased. I learned all this only many years later, after I'd grown up, left home, become a physician, had kids of my own. I'd tell her that none of it was her fault, it was just bad luck, but this didn't stop the pain or the tears that still flowed many decades later. The death of a child lasts a lifetime.

The origins of our careers, our life callings, are sometimes ascribed to chance or serendipity, but I believe that our paths are set more often, consciously or not, by highly meaningful events that shape our perceptions of who we are, how we fit into the fabric of existence, and that determine our motivations and goals.

Just as my mom had pursued a career in special ed to help other families like ours, my path was now set by a need to understand the origin of our family tragedy, decode this medical mystery, and perhaps prevent calamity from striking others. This wasn't a conscious plan, but was there nonetheless, gently simmering on a back burner of my mind. At so many points along the way, I'd find myself drawn back to Howard, Queens, and 1965. I needed to know more, to answer questions that may be unknowable, and to bring closure to the past.

CHAPTER 9

A Detour into Law

By the time junior year arrived, things seemed to be falling into place. My schoolwork was improving. And I found a great summer opportunity posted on the job board at Fordham University.*

"Busy Manhattan law firm seeks a highly motivated individual to help maintain a large library," it said. "Must be ambitious and a fast learner. Law students welcome to apply. Interested applicants should contact Ms. Dominique Brea at Fly, Shuebruk, Blume & Gaguine."

Perfect. Books I knew. I called the number and said that I was answering the ad. Oh my god, they're at Rockefeller Center! The office asked where I was calling from, and I said Fordham College, which was the truth. They told me to come up at 11:00 a.m. on Saturday for an interview with Ms. Brea.

I was determined to ace the interview. I visited the law library at NYU to get a feel for how it was organized, spent time thumbing through its massive card catalogue listing all of the books in the collection alphabetically and by topic, and walked around the stacks to understand how books and periodicals, both the popular ones in heavy use and those collecting dust, were stored. In the copier room, I asked a couple of students

* On weekends, I'd visit the local colleges, NYU, Fordham, and Queens College, and in the days before IDs were checked, I'd walk right into the student centers and peruse the summer job postings.

how they used the library, what worked and what didn't, and formulated a plan for my upcoming meeting.

I'd been to Rockefeller Plaza before, but only as a tourist to see the Christmas tree and skating rink in wintertime, sit in the audience of live television shows with Mom, and once to see the Rockettes down the street at Radio City Music Hall.* But I never knew what went on in the big majestic towers until that day, riding up the elevator at 45 Rockefeller Plaza, arriving at the 17th floor, and standing in front of the imposing double mahogany doors with the sign above that said Fly, Shuebruk, Blume & Gaguine, Attorneys at Law.

I entered the huge lobby, with its crystal clear windows looking down on the plaza and 5th Avenue. Immaculate. Three attractive secretaries at widely separated desks, each in front of a set of paired doors leading to the inner sanctums. One rose, greeting me with a smile.

"Welcome. Is it Mr. Hauser?"

"Yes, it's Steve; thank you."

"Ms. Brea will be with you shortly. Would you like a glass of water, coffee or tea, a soft drink?"

"Sure. Thanks. Do you have Pepsi?"

"Yes, indeed!" she answered with a smile, and disappeared behind one of the doors.

Toto, I've a feeling we're not in Flushing anymore.

And just then, Dominique Brea walked in. She looked like a Bond girl. Six feet tall, thin, elegant, perfect posture.

Thank goodness I wore my suit.

"Good afternoon. I'm Dominique Brea, executive assistant to attorneys Shuebruk and Blume. The other partners, Mr. Fly and Mr. Gaguine, are in our Washington offices. Thank you for contacting Fly, Shuebruk. May I call you Stephen?"

---

* Mom had a friend who was a Rockette, and she invited us to see the show.

A slight Euro accent, vaguely French with a British clip.

"Thank you; Steve is fine."

She led me down a long corridor, doors on both sides, each with the name of an associate, not yet a partner, then into a large open area where secretaries and various assistants worked at cubicles. At the very end was a spacious corner office, and we walked in.

"Stephen, please sit down." She pointed to a seat at the round conference table. Miraculously, a bottle of Pepsi was open and had been poured into a frosted glass half filled with ice. The fizz was still an inch high.

"You said that you called from Fordham. What year of law school are you in?"

"I'm sorry. I'm not in law school."

"Oh dear. We specifically posted the notice on the classifieds board at the Law School. The position is intended for a law student. Are you an undergraduate at Fordham?"

Clearly she had little experience with teens. I was 16 and looked even younger.

"No, ma'am; I'm in high school."

"Mr. Shuebruk specified that he wanted a law student. This is a complex job. Our law library is in disarray. Our attorneys must have ready access to books and documents that they need to prepare their casework. We require someone knowledgeable about the law to reorganize the library. I'm sorry."

My Pepsi was losing its fizz, and the frost on the glass was melting and beginning to resemble a relief map. I hesitated to drink but yielded to temptation. After a few gulps—and boy did that taste great—I responded. I was prepared for this.

"Ms. Brea, I understand books and libraries pretty well. Most important is that the library function efficiently for the users. The system of organization should be based on what works for them. If there are no strong preferences one way or the other, we could begin by cataloging the inventory with the Dewey Decimal System. The advantage here is that it is universally used, many people would be accustomed to it from their school libraries, and new volumes would automatically come with codes compatible with the system so they could easily be entered and stacked.

"The general code for law is 340–349. Fly, Shuebruk might have much of its content in categories 346 dealing with private law, 348 with regulations and cases, and 349 covering regional jurisdictions. Of course, some content would probably be in other areas, like government, social science, and economics, but these are easy to add.

"Do you know what system is used by the library in your Washington office? Ideally, we'd want to be in sync with them. Also, we could check with other outside libraries in Manhattan that the attorneys use. Do they use the Law Library of the New York City Bar?"

I got the job.

"The salary is one hundred twenty-five dollars per week. Is this satisfactory?"

"Yes, ma'am!" I pinched myself, trying not to faint. I was expecting maybe fifty dollars.

"Come; let me show you the library."

A chapel of jurisprudence. Mahogany everywhere. Floor-to-ceiling bookshelves, filled with stately leather-bound volumes, except for the windowed far wall decorated with small reading tables, swivel chairs, and green glass banker's lamps. In the center of the room, there was a large oval conference table, encircled by high-back leather chairs, and dominated by three large Tiffany-style glass lamps. Stray books everywhere, some open, others stacked, piled on floors, tables, chairs. More books than shelf space, this was for certain.

"There may be duplicates," I said, "or older editions that are out of date. We could store those somewhere else, or maybe give them away if no longer needed. And here, in this little area by the windows, we could separate out books that are used all the time, the essential ones. What do you think?"

"That would be perfect. I'll leave it up to you. Come with me; I'd like to introduce you to Mr. Shuebruk."

Tall, thin, patrician, Harvard educated, Peter Shuebruk greeted me with a smile, a handshake, and a warm welcome. And every day after that, usually in the morning or evening, he'd find time to stop by the library, ask me how I was doing, and speak of little things, the weather, the Yankees, or my future plans. He never spent more than a couple of minutes, but each second was consequential to me, because I was so honored to be in his presence.

And Dominique took me under her wing, making sure that I had everything I needed, even bringing me lunch each day. Small things that mean so much when you're just starting out in life. And when I'd bring my mint green Smith Corona portable typewriter from home, and index cards, rulers, and pens and pencils that I'd purchased at Woolworths, which was most days, she'd remind me again to just ask and they'd order whatever I needed. She also stressed the importance of professionalism.

"Our specialty is broadcast media, especially radio but also TV. Sometimes famous people will visit, and it is important that you be discreet and professional. You are representing Fly, Shuebruk. It is important to be well dressed every day because the partners may bring clients into the library. William F. Buckley was here just this morning."

Later that summer, I told Dominique that I needed three weeks off. I'd been accepted to an advanced placement biology course at Cornell University in Ithaca, New York. She smiled and hugged me.

"It's OK," she said.

I packed a year of growth into those 21 days at Cornell, along with 60 other aspiring seniors and even some real college students, all taking the same course. I was with really high achievers, and for the first time I felt that this was my group. We'd study hard, then hang out together playing basketball and spend late afternoons swimming at Cayuga Falls. Teenagers, finding our way in upstate New York in the summer of 1966.

When I returned to Fly, Shuebruk, my responsibilities expanded. They'd send me to Washington to deliver important files to the DC office or the FCC. And at the end of the summer, Peter Shuebruk called me to his office, thanked me for the work I'd done, and told me he wanted to give me a bonus, two weeks of salary. Maybe I could use it for college.

"We have a program that pays tuition for students who want to come to work with us after law school. I'm offering this to you should you decide to become a lawyer."

"Mr. Shuebruk, I am so grateful to you, everyone here, and especially to Dominique. And I'd love to keep working at Fly, Shuebruk. But I'm interested in science, and think I'd like to go to medical school."

CHAPTER 10

College Days

Walking across MIT's main courtyard on that first day, with its Doric columns, its great dome modeled on the Pantheon, and the names of scientists who had changed the world etched in large block letters in the limestone cornices of the grand buildings illuminated by a perfect blue sky, was a stirring experience. Behind me was the Charles River, with sailboats, footbridges, and the Boston skyline in the distance.

I thought I was at the center of the universe.

Science was on a roll. It had won World War II and cured polio. The space race was in full swing, front-page news most days, and everyone knew that science held the key to victory. MIT's provost, Jerome Wiesner, had been JFK's science advisor, and our Draper Laboratory was building computers and navigation systems that would soon be used by NASA to get to the moon. Science had become a national priority. The cold war would be won through technology. And at MIT, for the first time, German would no longer be required to graduate; American English was now the language of science.

During that memorable first week, as I struggled to understand special relativity in a class of ten, a student went up to the large blackboard at the front of the class and, with white chalk, scratched the main equations from memory, then proceeded to debate the professor about the best way to solve a particularly difficult variation.

The kid was 14 years old.

The rest of us looked on, amazed. I could always do math in my head and "see" equations, but this guy was in a whole different league. I wasn't intimidated, however; instead, I was proud to be in a class with someone so gifted. And when, after great effort and many weeks, I finally understood relativity—really understood it—the feeling of accomplishment was extraordinary. There is joy in figuring things out, and instilling this sense of excitement for discovery seemed to be the overarching goal of the undergraduate curriculum.* I was in my element and thrived as never before.

I made a mental note, however, to major in something other than physics and stay in a slower lane. One needs to be practical in life.

I pledged AEPi, my dad's fraternity at LSU. AEPi recruited freshmen not by boasting about its star athletes, as fraternities typically did, but by pointing to the fact that it had the highest grade point average on campus.

My first roommate at AEPi was Bill Rastetter, a charismatic guy with leading man looks and mythical energy. Whatever his goal—rowing, chemistry, or business, no matter—he'd lap the field. He spoke in near whispers, intimidating at close range.

We competed for the same girlfriend. He won, but we maintained a friendship that would carry through, decades later, to work that would change the face of brain disease research.

* * *

---

* Exams at MIT were open book, and students were bound to an honor system to attempt to solve the problems without seeking help from others. We often had three hours to complete final exams and were free to leave the classroom for library, home, or anywhere else. The answers were not found in books anyway, and rote memorization didn't help much—understanding the subject was what mattered.

It was 1968, there was widespread social unrest, and Boston was possibly the best place in the world to be if you were 18 and open to new ideas. I began the year as a young Republican and a supporter of the Vietnam War, like everyone else in my family, but by midyear had flipped 180 degrees.

I didn't get a haircut the entire year. I joined protests over the weaponry labs at MIT and campus visits of Dow Chemical Company, manufacturer of napalm. On the Sunday night radio show that I deejayed on MIT's local station, the politically neutral doo-wop of the fall term turned into lefty folk-rock by spring. I hung out at the sleep-ins at the MIT Student Center, where we sheltered an AWOL soldier and were entertained with music, theater, and giant screen showings of *Star Trek* and *Earth vs. the Flying Saucers*. We'd take breaks from the sanctuary to swim, play pickup basketball, or eat pizza and burgers and fries from the 24/7 fast food station in the building. And it all got even better when busloads of Wellesley girls disembarked, joining our sleep-in.

Boston wasn't perfect of course. Just under the surface lurked a particularly ugly strain of racism, more cloistered than in the Deep South but every bit as uncompromising. Black students were uncomfortable walking down Newbury Street, even more so going to Fenway Park, and a trip to Boston Garden to see the Bruins was out of the question. Yet somehow, even these flaws seemed fixable, and we were filled with optimism that our generation would repair society's ills, whether it was xenophobia, inequality, or war.

And as my horizons widened, the ties that bind began to fray. Family sacrifices everything to get you somewhere different, better, but when you get there, you become a different person. The memories of events that took place across nearly two decades, these remain, at least the important ones. But their emotional significance is now shared with other, more recent things: life with friends, the thrill of learning science, and new vistas.

* * *

I decided early on to major in chemistry at MIT, an easy call inspired by my earlier introduction to metallurgy at Brooklyn Tech. I was interested in the chemical composition of materials and was beyond fortunate that my first lab course in chemistry was taught by Dan Traficante. Dan's specialty was nuclear magnetic resonance (NMR) spectroscopy, a technique that measures perturbations in the movement of liquid-phase molecules in response to applied magnetic fields. By learning to read the pattern of signals recorded on the detector, one could decipher the atoms that comprise any small chemical compound, both inert ones and also biologic materials. Dan's passion for this area of chemistry was infectious, and interested students like me would spend long hours into the evening reviewing spectra with him, learning how to identify the chemical structures that each peak identified, and running additional samples to confirm and extend our results.

Exams were fantastic. We'd each be given a small vial containing a clear liquid with an unknown molecule dissolved in it, a different one for each student. We had a week to decipher the chemical structure, and the only rule was to do this by ourselves. An honor code, like everything else at MIT. Some patterns were tougher to interpret than others, but what really mattered was the process that we used rather than arriving at a perfect answer. It was basically a detective game, and even though each of our problems was different, the experience of being together with the other students, not in a classroom but in a lab, actively working on solutions, was enormous fun. As we sorted through the chemical bonds in our samples, we bonded as a group. Lasting friendships formed, and a big part of it was the tone that Dan set. It was a privilege to hang out with this crowd; they were curious about so many things, not only science.

Dan was a junior faculty member then, only in his mid-thirties. He had come from the Naval Academy, where he'd been an elite gymnast. Unlike most people at MIT, he'd talk to us about sports and exercise as much as chemistry. His New Joisey accent was vintage Joe Pesci. Darkly handsome, wiry, and with a motor that was always on. I learned early on that he was related to Santos Trafficante,* the Mafia kingpin who ran the Miami ports and is believed by some to have been behind JFK's assassination. Over time I became convinced that Dan knew more than he'd say about what actually happened to JFK, but I never summoned the courage to ask.

Dan taught us that a variation of NMR spectroscopy, first developed in the 1930s, could now be applied to solid materials as well, and that mining companies were already building machines to decipher the chemical constituents within mountains. The first images of a living organism were still a decade away, but Dan was convinced that his tool would one day revolutionize medicine. He was ahead of the curve in perceiving the future and was not shy about shouting it out, especially to medically minded undergraduates like me.

Indeed, down the road magnetic resonance imaging (MRI) would play a pivotal role in untangling multiple sclerosis. Dan's method would be adapted to visualize the nervous system noninvasively and in exceptional detail, providing a camera into the living brain. This would later allow us to track brain inflammation in people with MS over time and quantify the effect of interventions with far greater precision than possible with bedside

* There are numerous Anglicized spellings of the Trafficante surname, including Traficante and Traficant.

neurological exams. For the first time, we'd have a tool to efficiently test therapies against MS, and the clinical advances that followed would never have been possible without this foundational development.

* * *

We'd hear stories that Dan was competing with another Dan—Dan Kemp, the equally cool and even more popular organic chemistry professor. Possibly the most interesting guy on a campus filled with exceptionally interesting people.

Dan was MIT's version of Jay Gatsby. He had money and gave a lot of it away. He lived in a penthouse apartment with his cockatoo who'd wear sweaters that Dan knit by hand. He was an opera singer and Shakespearean actor, French cook and pastry chef, collector of exotic gems, a philosopher. And then he won the Massachusetts Lottery, proof that God doesn't distribute the fruits of the earth equally.

His teaching skills were legendary. MIT's formal lectures were held in "10–250," a huge amphitheater just off the Great Hall and main quadrangle of the campus. Nobelists could fill and command the 425-seat room, but junior faculty typically lectured to sparse crowds. Except for Dan. Beginning exactly on time, and armed with a portable microphone and a long stick of pristine white chalk, he'd start at the top left corner of the left section of the immense slate blackboard and trace the evolution of a set of pedagogic principles with a series of beautifully drawn chemical reactions and equations. As he wrote, he'd comment on the underlying science, perhaps the history of how the equations were deciphered, their utility for commercial products or medicines, and on occasion he'd sprinkle in a few digressions about the lives of students in the audience (how did he know that?), current events, or jokes.

There were no clocks in 10–250. At ten minutes before each

hour, a short horn would sound on the loudspeaker, and class would be over. Dan turned this endnote into theater. Just as he was completing the final line of the final symbol of the final reaction, perfectly sculpting the lower right corner of the giant blackboard, he'd signal the end of the lesson with a flourish, by dotting the last chemical symbol with an emphatic punctuation or waving his hand into the air. And at the same exact moment the horn would sound.

Dan was a pioneer in the field of protein folding, an area that would later prove key to understanding Alzheimer's and other neurodegenerative diseases. But it wasn't the details of his science that drew students in, it was his prowess as a teacher. There were many great scientists at MIT, but as an educator he had few peers.

CHAPTER 11

Being a Patient

Initially, it seemed like just the flu—nothing special, fever, sore throat, aches and pains. But unlike the flu, it didn't go away. It hit me just a few months after I'd arrived at MIT.

I called student health, explained the problem, and a nurse on the other end made an appointment for me. I arrived on time, said hi to the receptionist, and waited alone in a small antechamber outfitted with a couple of chairs. When the doctor came out, I was surprised to see that she was a woman, unusual in the 1960s. She walked toward me with a warm smile, placed her hand on my shoulder, and introduced herself as Dr. Sara Valenti. We walked together down a corridor to her office.

She motioned for me to sit in a chair, then sat down facing me. After a quick examination, she told me that my throat was red and tonsils and lymph nodes were swollen. My spleen was also enlarged, and this was the cause of my pain. Her tone was professional but sympathetic, a quality that also set her apart from many of the physicians I'd met. The next step, she told me, would be to obtain a few blood tests from the lab down the hall. These might reveal the cause, and she'd call as soon as the results were back. She looked me in the eye and touched my arm as she spoke. She seemed unhurried, and I had her undivided attention.

I hadn't even received a diagnosis, yet I felt comforted as I left the clinic. I had no guarantee that all was well—I just felt relief at knowing that someone who obviously cared was taking care of me. I was not alone, and this made all the difference.

* * *

The hallway phone rang in the fraternity house. An old black metal wall-mounted, rotary coin-operated phone that we learned to use only for incoming calls. Outgoing calls we'd make at the bank of pay phones located at the student center, or the BU women's dorm down the street, because we had a system, ritually passed on from one class to the next, to replace the coins with a hand-held tape recorder that would ping the sound of quarters and dimes dropping so that we wouldn't have to pay.

It was Dr. Valenti. Again, her tone was reassuring.

"Stephen, I wanted you to know that your blood tests have come back. They show that you have mono. Infectious mononucleosis. We think that it's caused by a virus. This is good news, because mono usually resolves within a few weeks. Can you come in to see me tomorrow morning at 9:00 a.m.?"

"Sure."

Everyone knew about mono, the "kissing disease." But given my social life at the time, there must be other ways to catch it. The next morning I hurried out of the fraternity house and motorcycled on my new Honda 90 to the student health center and her office.

"I'm so glad that we have an answer. How are you feeling?"

"Pretty bad, doctor. My throat is sore. But the worst part is that I'm so tired. I have no energy, food doesn't taste the same, and I'm sleeping a lot."

"These symptoms are all expected with mono. They'll stay with you for a couple of weeks at the least. Don't fight it. It's fine to stay in bed. You need rest. And whatever you do, please, no sports for the rest of the semester. This is the most important thing. You have an enlarged spleen that could rupture from even a mild injury."

Bad news, but I couldn't play anyway. I felt too sick, too tired. I moped around the fraternity house for a few days, but Christmas break and January open study month were coming up, so I decided to go home to Flushing, where Mom would take care of me.

Home cooking didn't seem to help much. I was exhausted, and sleep was my new best friend. I'd spend my waking hours plopped in a living room chaise, doing homework, watching TV, and picking at food delivered on a tray. After a couple of weeks, when nothing was better, Mom brought me to our family internist, who examined me, repeated the blood tests, and called back the next day.

"Your blood tests are all normal. The heterophile, which is the test for mono, is now negative. There's nothing wrong with you. Just go back to your normal life. No restrictions."

But I still felt awful. And when I returned to school in February, nothing had improved. I was horribly tired all the time. I wasn't depressed and wasn't trying to play hooky. I just felt sick.

So, I went back to the MIT clinic and was reunited with Dr. Valenti. My spleen was still enlarged but not as much as it had been, she said, and the tenderness was gone, which was a good sign. My lymph nodes were also now normal in size, and my bloodwork was "perfect."

"But why then am I still so tired?"

"Sometimes after a bad viral illness fatigue hangs on for a while. Take it day by day. Try to attend as many classes as you can, rest when you need to, and I'll keep in close touch with you. I'll be there to help."

The spring semester was a slog. I was sleeping far too much every day, forcing myself up in the morning, and depending on coffee to keep going. I reduced my class load. I read that there were two kinds of fatigue, "tiredness" and "brain fog." I had both. But I persevered, and in April or May the lassitude began to lift, and by June I was back to my old self.

I learned something from this experience. When you recover from an illness, you feel better than before you became sick. Maybe it is the joy of feeling well again. An unexpected dividend, something to look forward to when days are dark.

In retrospect, I probably had chronic fatigue syndrome,* the medical term for longstanding, unexplained fatigue. Some cases follow an infection, such as Epstein-Barr virus, but the true cause is unknown. Most physicians believe that chronic fatigue syndrome is not even a real medical illness at all—that it's all in the mind. But I know that it is real . . . because I had it.

Dr. Valenti was probably in her thirties then. Just starting out in medicine, in a role that many of her classmates likely judged as lower rung, a junior frontline physician at a quiet student health clinic, diagnosing mostly benign conditions while triaging the few serious ones to experts at the elite Boston hospitals across the river. But to me she was a great physician. Like Counselor Dave a decade earlier, she excelled in the "care" part of "healthcare"—not only treating the illness but also caring for the person. Managing the illness is often the easy part. Taking care of people as individuals is far more challenging, and vastly more time-consuming. The difficulties are largely emotional, the sum of person after person, family after family, looking for help and not realizing, or being able to accept, that sometimes little can be done. My mono was self-limited and would improve on its own, but many maladies at the time were untreatable and incurable.

Still, I knew that I wanted to be like Dr. Valenti.

---

* Recently renamed myalgic encephalomyelitis, this condition has had many monikers but few scientific leads.

CHAPTER 12

Foundations

"I've never seen Francis Crick in a modest mood" is how James Watson's sizzling bestseller *The Double Helix* begins.

One benefit of being sick was that I had time to read, and it was during this break that I encountered a book that would change the course of my career.

The Double Helix was Watson's tale of his discovery of DNA, the substance of heredity, when he was a 23-year-old trainee working in Crick's lab in Cambridge, England. What made the book stupendous was not just the science, although the science was the discovery of the century, but also the odd characters, high ambition, and wild intrigue. It made science sexy and even more exciting than I'd imagined. I was determined to study DNA. Here was the secret of life, and maybe the answer to disease.

So when junior year arrived and it came time to select a scientific mentor, I chose Har Gobind Khorana, a soft-spoken Indian biochemist working in this new field of molecular genetics. Khorana had already won a Nobel Prize for his role in cracking the genetic code, revealing how the sequence of DNA building blocks specifies the assembly of proteins from amino acids.* Watson and Crick discovered the structure of genes, but

---

* DNA building blocks come in four flavors—A, T, C, and G—and the sequence of

Khorana opened a window into how genes work.* Essentially everything that we know about genetics today, including genetic diagnosis and even gene therapy, followed from this discovery.

I cold-called Khorana one afternoon, and he accepted me on the spot. I think that he just wanted to help a motivated undergraduate student and assumed that there was a reasonable chance I'd be useful. Anyway, MIT was that sort of place. He invited me to meet him the next day in his large wood-paneled office, decorated with an enormous sculpture of the RNA molecule that he'd recently chemically synthesized, the first artificial gene ever made. I was dazzled to be face-to-face with this living legend. It was lunchtime, and he offered me half of his sandwich, telling me to just lean over his desk while eating. I was careful not to leave crumbs.

Located in a large wing off the left arm of the Great Court, Khorana's laboratory teemed with young people, men and women in long white lab coats, scuttering between shared refrigerated rooms, where reagents were stored and experiments carried out, and room-temperature labs with huge chemical hoods against the walls, where dense shielding offered protection from the highly radioactive substances used to mark the chemical building blocks that were being slowly and painstakingly synthesized into genetic material, DNA and RNA, using the arduous methods of the day.

Most everyone spoke with an accent, ambitious young scientists-in-training who'd come from all corners of the world for the honor of working with Khorana. Publishing a scientific paper with the master would be career-defining. Most would

---

three DNA molecules in a row specifies which of the 20 amino acids is next assembled into a protein chain.

* Khorana shared the 1968 Nobel Prize in Physiology and Medicine with Marshall Holley and Joshua Nirenberg for this work.

return to their native countries, but the truly talented and fortunate few might secure faculty positions in the United States. The big event was the weekly lab meeting, where work in progress would be presented by one member of the group, and then sharply critiqued by the others, who'd run up to the chalkboard to sketch out alternative conclusions to explain the data or develop ideas for new experiments. It seemed like a free-for-all, but it wasn't. It was controlled mayhem, a cauldron of creativity, and the ultimate meritocracy.

Khorana was the ringmaster. He was clearly shooting for a second Nobel, they'd whisper, a feat that at the time had been accomplished by only one other person, Marie Curie. This one would be for synthesizing genes, the molecules of life. I'd see him working at the bench alongside his trainees, in the same white coat, mouth pipetting the dangerous liquid by sucking it into a transparent tube, carefully observing its upper level to avoid ingesting any, and hoping not to cough, or worse yet, hiccup. Everyone knew that no matter how many other demands were on Khorana's time he'd remain a hands-on working scientist who mastered every technique used in his lab. He walked the walk, and this was a big part of what made him so admired. But most important was the work itself, and the ideas. Conversations in the lab centered on synthesizing genes from scratch, developing ways to do this more rapidly,* understanding life, creating life.

This was far more exciting than any science fiction I'd consumed as a kid.

Khorana sent me to his lieutenant, Uttam (Tom) RajBhan-

* In a famous conclusion to a 1971 paper, Khorana outlined the polymerase chain reaction (PCR) method that would later change the face of molecular biology and make the cloning of genes feasible and widespread.

dary,[*] an affable chemist from Nepal, who designated me for assignment down the pecking order to a team of two, a male postdoctoral fellow and his female technical assistant. What a team they were. They had arrived at MIT together about 18 months earlier. He'd been studying to be a priest, but then he met her, a beautiful nun. They fell in love, left the Church, and became scientists. They were a captivating pair, charismatic extroverts. After work we'd sometimes go out for spicy Szechuan food and wind up in a coffeehouse. They'd talk about growing up in the rural Midwest, joining the Catholic Church, discovering each other at the convent. But even more interesting was the story of how they escaped, were excommunicated, and reborn as chemists. Under their wing, I worked for the next year helping to decipher and then synthesize from scratch the building blocks of a second RNA molecule. The first had already been memorialized as sculpture in Khorana's office. The project was trailblazing, yet I wasn't as engaged as I might've been. I loved the idea of synthesizing the chemicals of life, but the day-to-day experiments, the mixing and measuring and reacting of chemicals in test tubes, were too dry for my taste. I needed work that connected more directly with people and their problems. I wanted to help people like my childhood friend Robert and most of all like my brother Howard. I wasn't cut out to be a basic scientist, but if I could use the science to study real health problems, then I knew the work would grab and sustain me.

* * *

Now committed to a career in medicine, my biology courses would be particularly important. Our core biology course was

---

* Tom RajBhandary grew up in the valley of Kathmandu. See "A Conversation with Uttam RajBhandary," MIT Department of Biology, available on YouTube.

taught by Salvador Luria, another illustrious figure at MIT. Luria left Italy before World War II, after Mussolini banned Jews from receiving research fellowships. He moved to Paris, then narrowly escaped by bicycle as the invading Nazi forces approached. He made it to the south of France, and in Marseille secured a visa and safe passage to the United States. Now, more than two decades later, he was about to lose his federal research grants again, this time not because of his ancestry but because of his opposition to the war in Vietnam. Fortunately for him, he'd soon receive positive news from the Nobel Prize Committee and could now secure research funding from other, less partisan, sources.

Outside of the classroom we'd see Luria lunching at the student center, at a table with other MIT superstars. We were in awe of them, and I had to work hard not to stare. Philip Morrison, the polio-riddled physicist who'd helped construct and even loaded the nuclear weapon on the *Enola Gay* as it was headed for Hiroshima. Jerome Lettvin, a pioneer in understanding how the brain sees, husband to his equally famous wife Maggie, a fitness instructor and PBS celebrity. Another regular at the table was Noam Chomsky, a god in the field of linguistics, a social critic and political activist, and one of several MIT faculty honored with a place on Nixon's official enemies list. Sometimes they'd be joined by another name on that list, Jerome Wiesner, who evolved from cold warrior in the Kennedy administration to staunch advocate for arms control.

The 1960s was a period when power and expertise of all kinds came under attack, and science was no exception, but we felt incredibly fortunate to learn in and out of the classroom from this group of polymaths. So different in their interests and politics and personal styles, they were united in being supremely accomplished. For the 20-year-olds like me in their midst, they radiated a subliminal message: science is a wonderfully tolerant and highly social enterprise, but the price of admission is high. One needs to make a big difference in the world.

One area in which biology was making a big difference in those days was viruses. The development of effective vaccines against the dreaded poliovirus in the 1950s turned virologists into public figures; Salk and Sabin became household names. By the late 1960s, advances in cell biology and genetics had led to an explosion in new knowledge and optimism that other viral scourges, including viruses implicated in cancer, might soon be wiped out, just as polio had been.

Luria was one of the world's foremost experts on viruses. He'd written the classic book on the subject. One memorable lecture was on herpes viruses. I learned that they cause many human illnesses—chickenpox and shingles and cold sores—and that another family member was the virus that struck my mom's friend Janet back in Springfield Court. But the most phenomenal revelation was a new discovery—infectious mononucleosis was also caused by a herpes virus, named for its discoverers, Epstein and Barr. The Epstein-Barr virus or EBV.

Talk about hitting close to home! I raced to the library to read a few papers. I learned that mono is caused by a prolonged infection with Epstein-Barr, producing a powerful immune response against the virus. It's like a very bad flu, but longer lasting. Some symptoms are caused by the virus itself, but others are probably due to the body's attempt to fight back. I was sick from friendly fire. My immune system had become overactive.

Amazingly, EBV infections in infancy and childhood usually produce few or no symptoms but on occasion can cause a cancer of the immune system known as lymphoma. On the other hand, when infection is delayed until adolescence, as in my case, then the typical symptoms of infectious mono appear. Delayed infection with EBV is more common in developed societies, areas where mono is also prevalent. Maybe our modern focus on cleanliness and hygiene isn't always a good thing; the immune system wasn't designed for a later-life encounter with Epstein-Barr.

Luria also taught us that once these viruses infect a host, they can hide, dormant, for the rest of their time on earth. They are perfect invaders. They start by infecting cells in many different areas of the body but then retreat to isolated, secluded hideouts. And there they remain, protected, for the long term, inside just a few cells. This makes it extraordinarily difficult to flush out these tiny beasts, or develop vaccines against them. Or understand if they are responsible for other long-lasting problems of immune overactivity, not only the chronic fatigue of mono but maybe other illnesses, autoimmune diseases . . . even MS.

* * *

Shortly after arriving at MIT, I was walking down the main corridor and passed a door with an overhead sign that read "Upward Bound," which turned out to be a big brother, big sister program for inner-city teens. I walked in, and began a relationship that I'd maintain throughout my college years.

My first charge was Carl, a kid from Cambridge Rindge and Latin School who was oriented toward math and science and had a ready stream of words and a quick wit. He struck me as a natural leader, and he'd speak to me of sky-high ambitions—get into one of the Ivies or MIT, get a doctorate.

We'd work together two afternoons each week, usually at MIT. Sometimes he'd come back with me to my fraternity house for dinner. I thought that his prospects for success were outstanding—that is until I visited his home, a cramped, rundown apartment in the central Cambridge projects, in those days a dangerous neighborhood. Carl had no father, and to make ends meet, his mom worked both day and night jobs. His grandmother would make dinner for the family and help Carl and his two younger sisters with their homework as best she could. But most of the time Carl was pretty much on his own. He also had a history of getting into trouble, although nothing thus far that seemed too serious. A few playground fights, a bag of stolen candy.

Each spring, we geared up for the summer session of Upward Bound, an intensive six-week sleepaway camp at nearby Wellesley College. I worked with the other counselors, all students at MIT or Wellesley, to prepare a packed schedule of morning classes; afternoons were spent reading, swimming, boating on the lake, and playing sports.

We'd take over several college dorms, eat, sleep, and live together. It was an immersive, 24/7 experience, and we bonded in ways that we never could during the busy winter months. Here I became even closer to Carl; he'd say that I was his brother, that we'd be friends for life. I taught science and math, and also ran the Wellesley College observatory, where during one of our evening astronomy sessions we watched the moon landing of Apollo 11.

It was a Sunday evening, and I'd invited as a guest speaker Charles Stark Draper, the MIT professor who developed the navigation system that made the moon trip possible. Draper arrived in a classy green Jaguar racecar wearing a jaunty Irish flatcap. And there, under the starlight of the hilltop observatory, dome open to the heavens, gazing in turn at the details of the lunar landscape through the eyepiece of the giant 24-inch telescope, knowing that at just that moment two human beings were actually walking on the moon, Doc Draper regaled us with stories of boyhood dreams of space travel, the science behind the moon landing, and what it would take for the Apollo 11 astronauts to return home safely.

Afterward, the other counselors would say "That was phenomenal! How in the world did you get Doc Draper here?" They assumed that I had some special relationship and were incredulous to learn that I'd just cold-called with an invitation and that he'd accepted on the spot. A lesson in generosity.

We made progress at Upward Bound—none of our charges dropped out—but we still had a long way to go. I'd soon learn just how far.

In my senior year I walked into the Upward Bound office one morning to check in. Mike Efron, who led the program from its earliest days, ran out of his office to meet me. Tears were in his eyes.

"Steve, Carl was shot last night. He died before anyone could call for help. I was over to his house this morning. The funeral is later this week."

He didn't even make it to his 20th birthday, a victim of the pitfalls that our program was designed to avoid. A gang-related shooting and a drug deal gone bad. I'd tutored him for more than two years. We spent so much time together, but I had no inkling that drugs or gangs had entered his life. There were clues, but I didn't connect the dots. The kid just needed one or two more breaks in life to tip the scales in the other direction.*

* * *

My closest friend and roommate at AEPi was Alan Brown, an ROTC Navy guy and ocean engineering major from a very blue-collar family in New Bedford. You could hear his Southie accent from miles away. We had three things in common: we loved baseball, rock and roll music, and MIT.

In our senior year we moved to an off-campus apartment with two other fraternity brothers. Terry was a soft-spoken, laid-

---

* Just a few years later, another kid from Cambridge Rindge and Latin would join the MIT Upward Bound program, a gangly kid who'd recently moved to Cambridge from Kingston, Jamaica. This youngster, named Patrick Ewing, had an advantage that Carl did not. Patrick was seven feet tall and athletically gifted; he'd go on to a storied career in professional basketball.

back iconoclast with long, curly, black afro-style hair, bushy black beard, and thick black eyeglasses. Always smiling, the spitting image of Jerry Garcia. He was a Jewish kid from the northeast, but soon after moving in went to Cambridge City Hall and changed his legal name to Wong. His parents threatened to disinherit him if he carried this out, but he did it anyway: "I've always respected Chinese culture. I love Chinese food. I'd like to open a Chinese restaurant someday, and this makes it seem more authentic."

Our other new roomie, named Steve like me, was an MIT student who only wanted to be a biker, like Dennis Hopper in *Easy Rider* or Marlon Brando in *The Wild One*. Ruggedly handsome and athletic, Steve majored in motorcycle stunts, generally performed in the middle of the night on the public streets of Cambridge, after which he'd return to the apartment to party with his collection of biker girlfriends.

Somehow, in this chaos of our own making, Alan and I remained lasered in on our schoolwork, goals, and future. The tumult around us only improved our focus.

Science, like other creative activities, challenges us to see the world in new and unexpected ways. It favors those who are open to different ways of thinking and who delight in challenging established ideas. Scientists are often eccentrics, and they seek out other nontraditional people, mavericks, norm violators. Unusual people and unusual ideas. Offbeat was run of the mill here, and there was no such thing as odd. It felt just like home . . . but with supercharged learning. And I thrived as I never could have imagined.

CHAPTER 13

The Seeds of a Career

My experiences at MIT only strengthened my wish to become a physician. I'd have chosen medical school even without the incentive of an automatic draft deferment for medical students, although this was certainly a bonus. I'd lost the draft lottery, broadcast on prime-time TV, so a one-way ticket to Vietnam was waiting. Fortunately, I had an alternative. In my senior year an envelope arrived from Harvard Medical School with news that I'd been accepted to the class of 1975.

My mom said that even the rabbi was happy. In the Jewish religion, life begins when the fetus is accepted to medical school.

The medical school was located three miles south of Harvard Square and Harvard's main campus, within walking distance of MIT's fraternity row, a straight shot up Boylston Street, past Fenway Park on the left and a massive Sears department store on the right.

The school was a permanent construction zone, but there was still enough left of its original stately 19th-century limestone-and-brick campus that we could live happily within its confines and mostly forget that a gigantic biomedical complex surrounded us.

On sunny days, we'd stretch out on the grassy courtyards and quiet gardens not yet gobbled up by the concrete-and-steel high-rise buildings housing patients, laboratories, and research facilities. The ever-expanding complex embodied the transformation that was changing the face of medicine, away from the neighborhood family doctor who'd visit you at home and knew the names of your kids to a "provider" who records work units earned and is under the thumb of executives at giant healthcare conglomerates. This new system was soulless, but it produced major benefits: real medical advances and higher standards of care. However, it also made it more difficult for physicians to develop the kind of relationships with patients that made medicine so rewarding in the first place. And as medicine evolved in complexity, it was also becoming more daunting and confusing to patients. A personal touch was more important than ever; indeed, it would always be the soul of the profession.

Fortunately, Harvard Medical School had in its own way become more patient focused. A new curriculum reduced time spent in passive classroom learning and brought us into contact with real patients in our first semester. Women were also joining the ranks of medical students, not yet in equal numbers, and there were still barriers in macho specialties like orthopedics and surgery, but the school was beginning to look like a coed campus. And permeating our mindset was a belief that we'd soon have the necessary tools to solve health problems that had plagued humanity since ancient times. A revolution was brewing, and we wanted to be in on the action.

* * *

I told everyone that I wanted to be a general internist, but from day one I sought out the neurologists—not necessarily to become one, but to understand cognitive disabilities, a link to my brother Howard's illness and the mentally and physically handicapped children my mom taught. I arranged to spend a year in child neurology with Bob DeLong, a dedicated teacher and superb physician who led the service at the Massachusetts General Hospital. Bob had a lifelong interest in autistic children with special talents.

Some people on the autistic spectrum have accomplished great things. Isaac Newton, Alan Turing, and Nikola Tesla are examples from science, and in the arts, Glenn Gould and Tim Burton qualify. But the kids I studied under Bob were in a different universe. They weren't headed for success, but their unusual skills were even more interesting to me precisely because they were of very little benefit.

Each week I'd meet with one child, usually accompanied by the mother and sometimes father or siblings. Bob would start each day off by introducing me to the family. He'd ask how the child was doing at home, review medications, benefits and side effects, then leave them in my care for the day. I'd get the medical history. It was a fabulous learning experience.

The mothers would recount the story of the pregnancy, early weeks of life, and that traumatic moment when they first knew that all was not OK. At this point, you'd see them experience the power of their loss in a grimace or a pause as they wrestled with the painful nagging doubt about whether they had done anything to cause the problem. They'd gone over it in their minds, again and again, searching for clues to the cause of the tragedy. My mom had done the same thing, and to this day believes she was to blame for bringing a damaged child into the world.

The mother would bring a favorite pacifier or trinket needed to keep the child calm: a pillow, rag doll, or blocks to line up in rows, a favorite cookie or drink. We'd sit together on the floor, and I'd offer the special items as distractions while I attempted to perform a neurological exam. I'd jot down the rare words, describe the child's behavior and activities, record mood, anxiety, tantrums, and assess vision, strength, sensation, coordination, and gait. But mostly I'd just hang out with the child: observing, playing—severe autistics don't really play, so I'd mostly place an object, or sometimes myself, in their line of sight to see what happened—and try to bring out any unusual proclivities.

The kids were mostly unknowable. But I'd get to know the mothers, sometimes the fathers also. They'd often ask what sparked my interest in autism and youngsters like their child, and I'd tell them about my brother, how his illness affected my family, and my mom's career in special ed. Sometimes they'd ask what caused their child to be autistic. By now I was confident enough to say that autism was as real a biologic problem as any other brain illness. It had nothing to do with parenting. I'd say that many different diseases could produce autism, but the common denominator was injury to particular parts of the brain—damage to the social circuits.

Near the end of the day Bob DeLong would return, and in 15 minutes I'd learn more than I had in the previous five hours. One little boy had a diet dominated by animal crackers. He'd only eat other foods if animal crackers were also offered. Bob lined up the little cookies, checkerboard style, on the play table. The tyke lunged for them, slurping up the cookies one by one.

"Watch this," DeLong told me, "he's missed a couple of cookies in the upper right corner of the table. It happens every time. He neglects that part of his visual field. He can see it, but objects there don't catch his attention. The optic radiations for the right superior visual field travel through the left temporal lobe. His visual neglect is a sign of left temporal lobe disease."

"Watch closely when he's playing," Bob said with another child. "He always reaches with his left hand. He's a lefty. Most autistic children are. But look at his right hand. Can you see how he's tightly grasping his thumb? That's not normal. It's called a cortical thumb. Now let's watch him walk across the room," he continued. "Can you see how his right arm swings less than the left? These are all signs of a left hemisphere injury."

Here I saw, time and again, lovely, loving parents who'd have done anything to help their children. And I saw how deeply the mothers suffered. Their kids gave nothing back. No eye contact, no recognition. Bring them toward you and they'd kick or punch or spit; leave them alone and they'd go into a corner to line up blocks, chairs, spoons, whatever was there, in long rows. Disturb the rows and they'd fly into a frenzy, flap their hands, blink, rock back and forth, bang their head against the wall, screech or bark, make clacking sounds but no real words. There was often no sign that they recognized words at all, or that they had a need for any sort of communication with others.

But it was their amazing skills that really drew DeLong and me to these youngsters. Talents that revealed enormous underlying brainpower. Although this feature of autism had been recognized since the early 20th century, its biological basis was entirely unknown. How could such impaired children have these special gifts?

One four-year-old would read the *New York Times* out loud, cover to cover, every day, all day long. That kid loved the *New York Times*, but it was impossible to determine that anything he was reading made sense to him. And save for the nonstop reciting, he was totally noncommunicative.

"Jimmy, come here. I'd like to show you something really neat," I'd say. But he just kept reading aloud.

"Spiro Agnew, the vice president of the United States has been dealing with charges of tax evasion and receiving bribes," he'd say. "President Richard Nixon expressed full support for his beleaguered vice president and stated that resignation had not been considered."

I'd try again: "Jimmy, I have a present for you. Come look at this beautiful red fire truck."

No response. His mother would then take a marshmallow out of his lunch box. It was his favorite food, and the only stimulus that could distract him from his recital.

Another little guy knew the calendar trick. Just ask him for any date, say, March 17, 2054, and the kid would immediately blurt out the correct day of the week, "Tuesday," but otherwise he was silent.

I met a pint-sized math whiz. He could remember long lists of numbers and calculate up to a dozen digits in his head.

There was a little girl who was an artist. She'd draw beautiful pictures of her home, family, landscapes, but she, too, had no language or interest in others. She'd only engage with her parents when they offered her crayons or writing paper. Take them away, perhaps for mealtime, and she'd go bananas.

I was drawn to them. I also recognized some of me and others I knew in these kids, especially the memory wizards. I used to do similar tricks—mine weren't as good, but they were still reasonably amusing. As a kid, I knew every major league baseball player's batting average, and could recite the artist, label, year, and sometimes month of release of many early rock songs. A good memory is very useful but remembering too much might sometimes be a bad thing.

The most important lesson was that to really understand autism, I had to see it—a lot of it—in person. Book learning was inadequate. Much of the medical literature at the time ascribed autism to mothers who were cold and aloof, who didn't hold their infants close to their bodies. This was not only wrong, it was cruel. Over a full year of meeting with mothers, not one fit this description. It was known that many different factors can lead to autism, such as intrauterine infections, impaired supply of blood, oxygen, or glucose to the brain, as well as a host of genetic disorders.

There are so many pathways to autism, but the similarities in behavior of the children he'd studied convinced Bob DeLong that there must be a common site in the brain where the injury occurs.

At the time, almost nothing was known about what actually happened in the brains of these children. Most autism researchers were psychologists, skilled in family dynamics but uninterested in neuropathology. That's where we came in.

The most beautiful scientific experiments are the simple ones, and Bob had chosen for me a magnificently simple yet terribly important project. I was to learn brain anatomy and identify changes that cause autism. Bob's earlier research had already shaped the general outline of the story. Some of these youngsters had damage in their temporal lobe, the part of the brain adjacent to the ears, and he theorized that autism might reside here, especially on the left side where language is known to live.* My job was to study the brain tissue of autistic children who had died, and the brain X-rays of our autistic patients, to test, develop, and refine his theory.

I spent time digging into examples of known temporal lobe damage, one in monkeys and another in humans. Klüver-Bucy syndrome was named after the two scientists who first performed, or perpetrated, surgery to remove the anterior temporal lobes from healthy monkeys. After surgery, the animals superficially seemed fine. Strong, well-coordinated, normal vision. But when returned to the colony, they no longer had any interest in other monkeys. They'd perch in a corner, alone, silent, repetitively handling things, even dangerous things like snakes that monkeys normally avoid. They couldn't distinguish dangerous from safe. They had monkey autism.

---

* In right-handers; in lefties, language can live on either side but is often distributed across both hemispheres.

Bob DeLong also encouraged me to learn about a temporal lobe disease in adults, encephalitis* caused by infection with the herpes simplex virus. Herpes simplex attacks the temporal lobes. When it severely injures the left side but only slightly damages the right, the victims lose their ability to understand language and show no interest in others.†

"Imagine," Bob DeLong would say, "what it would be like if herpes encephalitis struck newborns. I'll bet that they'd grow up to look autistic."

His comment hit home.

"Dr. DeLong," I replied, "even when it strikes adults, I think that something like autism could result."

Although I didn't have a name for it then, encephalitis had been in my thoughts since I was six or seven years old. This was the illness that had turned Mom's closest friend Janet from a social butterfly into a recluse. Janet's condition was eerily similar to what I'd seen in severely autistic children, and my interest in temporal lobe disease intensified. I now went to work with stored brain tissue from autistic children, donated by their parents to our hospital in the hope that other kids might someday be helped through research. We examined every part of the brain and, just as Bob predicted, found temporal lobe disease, mostly on the left side—not in every case, but often enough to be convincing. We then turned to brain X-rays from living autistic children, a primitive technique by today's standards, but one offering a hazy view, just a glance, into the center of the temporal lobes.‡ It was

* "Encephalitis" refers to an inflammation of the brain; most cases are due to an infection or autoimmune process.

† Lose both sides completely, and patients may not recover at all, or they may appear vegetative.

‡ As young neurologists, we became expert at performing pneumoencephalography or PEG, a test involving injection of air into the spinal fluid and then sitting the patient upright so that the air rises to the head, visualizing the ventricles, or lakes, in the center of the cerebral hemispheres. PEGs are intensely painful, but a number of our autistic children registered no apparent pain during the procedure. Soon, far more

enough to confirm consistent damage to this area. Wow! We'd discovered something important and proceeded to write a scientific paper, my first, describing our findings.*

* * *

I needed a job to stay afloat, even in medical school. I wasn't yet a real doctor, but now had some bona fide medical skills, including special expertise in childhood brain disorders.

So I became a contract employee for the State of Massachusetts. On weekend mornings, a small van would appear in front of our dorm and transport a half dozen medical students to one of the state-run custodial institutions across Massachusetts. There we'd review, summarize, and interpret the often-shoddy medical records of the patients. Most had stopped taking new patients, but hundreds of people who'd been admitted in decades past still lived there. Some were now octogenarians who'd been deposited at the door as infants without any information about their past or family. I'd later learn that much of our cataloging was in preparation for a state effort to consolidate the institutions and ultimately close them down.

I was usually assigned to Belchertown State Hospital for the Feeble-Minded, a sad place in a beautiful part of western Massachusetts. Dickens would have been hard-pressed to imagine a bleaker name, which harkened back to an earlier era and a more callous attitude toward people with intellectual disabilities. Though it was now the 1970s, the name still held. I'd spend most of the day summarizing medical records, but always made time to visit with the people whose histories I'd reviewed.

---

accurate and painless imaging tests such as MRIs would replace PEGs for diagnosis of most brain conditions.

* "Temporal Lobe Findings in Early Infantile Autism," published in the journal *Brain* in 1975.

I'd reach them by wandering down long, dark, windowless corridors, past bolted double-door entryways requiring latchkeys to pass through, to the pod of rooms where the residents lived.

An aide would buzz me in. There was a cot in each room, sometimes a chair and table, but little else. Many residents were bedbound, and some had not been outdoors for decades. By this time I was pretty well accustomed to the terribly sad conditions that disabled people sometimes face, but the sights I witnessed in those backrooms at Belchertown stung as few things would again. I met an alert, talkative woman* with profound congenital hydrocephalus, a blockage of the water-filled ventricles in the brain, whose head had expanded to the size of a beachball; two aides were required to gently rotate her head from one side to the other, a daily routine to protect against bedsores of the scalp. And an older man who spent his days strapped in a chair, moaning, swatting away imaginary bugs, limbs in constant motion, the side effect of medications used to control his hallucinations. The conditions were worse than deplorable, but many residents were so impaired that it was difficult to imagine how the institution could do much better. I now understood why my parents had been so adamant about caring for my brother at home.

Most of the patients at Belchertown were born with terrible disabilities, exactly like my brother. But others had been normal until something catastrophic destroyed their brain—encephalitis, syphilis, or brain trauma.

The most shocking cases were those of children who may have been normal—we couldn't tell for sure from the records—but had been admitted because there was no other place for

* She was only able to speak simple pleasantries such as "Hello!", "How are you?", and "What a lovely day!" even when it was raining outside.

them to go. After decades of life in an impoverished environment, where nothing is taught and little expected, they became institutionally retarded. Real-life evidence of the critical role of environment in shaping how our brains work.

CHAPTER 14

Reaching Closure

By now I had come to understand early life brain injuries pretty well, not just autism but also other forms of mental and physical disability—including Howard's. I was ready to examine his past as best I could. I'd try to find answers, not that they'd bring him back to life, but maybe the knowledge could help my parents move beyond their sadness. I was still only a medical student, by no means an expert neurologist, not even a real doctor yet, but I'd absorbed much, and with the overconfidence of youth felt equipped to crack this mystery that had haunted me for so long.

The first step in neurologic diagnoses is to decide where the problem is in the nervous system; only after figuring out the anatomy can the cause—what the problem is—be understood. I needed to go back in time and reconstruct a neurologic examination on my brother. His vision was excellent: he could see me from far away, he'd laugh as I approached, and when he saw that I was bringing one of his favorite things, a toy or ice cream, he'd begin crawling to me, laughing. His eyes appeared normal and moved smoothly, a memory confirmed by old photos. And he loved when I whispered songs in his ear, silly songs like "Abba Dabba Dabba." This means that large areas of Howard's brain were working normally—the visual nervous system originating just behind his eyes and traveling deep in the hemispheres, all the way to the back of the brain, the occipital lobes. And normal eye movements and hearing meant that the brain stem just below the hemispheres was mostly intact.

My brother's most obvious neurologic symptoms were severe cognitive and motor incapacities. At nearly eight years old he'd not acquired language—he couldn't speak, and didn't understand words. He could crawl but not walk, and could grab things with his fists but had no control of individual finger movements. And he was completely incontinent. Sensation was tougher to reconstruct; Howard would cry when he hurt himself, but often he'd bang his head repetitively against hard surfaces—walls or radiators—and his room had to be padded and child-proofed to prevent injuries.

Language lives in the middle (parietal and temporal) lobes of the brain, in the left hemisphere in right-handers, but in lefties like my brother it's more likely located on both sides.* Motor function is in the rear of the frontal lobes, with sensation just behind that. And cognitive loss can be more diffusely represented, with greater retardation indicating more global damage. So I was developing a model of the anatomy of my brother's brain damage. Large areas of injury must have existed across both cerebral hemispheres, especially in the posterior frontal and parietal-temporal regions, but the brain stem and spinal cord had been spared.

Having now developed an anatomic model of my brother's disability, I was ready to consider the cause. My brother was severely retarded, both mentally and physically. I knew that many cases of mild retardation arise in families who start off

---

* Handedness is controlled by the contralateral (opposite) hemisphere, also the side where speech and some other cognitive activities reside. Right-handed people—94 percent of the population—are usually left-brain dominant. If the left side of the brain is injured early in life, then these functions can move to the right hemisphere, and the brain injury results in left-handedness later in life. This is why many mentally impaired people are left-handed.

at the lower end of the intellectual bell curve; these are caused by an unlucky draw when the genes are handed out. Profound retardation, on the other hand, usually results from genetic mutations or catastrophic brain injuries—say, a virus or stroke during gestation or early life. This was the most likely category for my brother.

Howard was a normal-looking child, without any of the deformities that so often accompany genetic illnesses. And there was no history of other children in our family with similar problems, which would also have pointed to a genetic problem. The only feature that suggested a genetic cause were his frequent infections, with those sky-high fevers, and his difficulty in fighting these off. This could reflect an inherited immune deficiency of some kind, but might just as likely be explained by pneumonias caused by aspiration of food particles into the lungs because his damaged brain left him unable to swallow normally.

I read everything available about genetic causes of immune deficiency and pored over picture books showing the abnormal faces of children born with constellations of immune and nervous system problems. None resembled my brother.

I needed more history. As painful as this would be, I had to revisit the nightmare of Howard's birth with my parents. I knew that it was still a deep wound that had not healed, especially for my mom, but I had no choice. This would be the last best chance to reach closure. I learned that at the beginning of life, he'd been dusky, clinging to life, so something very bad had happened around the time of birth.

When I next returned to New York, I sat down with my folks and my brother David. For the first time, I saw them look at me first as a physician—which I wasn't yet of course—instead of their son or brother. A transition had taken place.

"Mom, what do you remember from the hospital? You said that someone told you that Howard had been dropped at birth."

"I can't remember exactly. Maybe a nurse said this later on, when I was walking in the hallway. Maybe she wasn't a nurse, she might have been a housekeeper. She might have said that it's possible he could have been dropped. I'm really not sure."

My dad chimed in. "I don't think anything bad happened in the delivery room. They said his color was dusky, he was lifeless, he wasn't breathing. The doctor said that sometimes this happens when the umbilical cord is wrapped around the neck, but this wasn't the case with Howard."

I pressed on. "Mom, you've told me that there might have been a problem in the heart or the lungs."

"This is what I heard but the doctors really didn't know," she said. "They knew so little back then."

So often it's the history that's wrong. A lesson that I tell medical students every day.

My mom had assumed that Howard had been dropped at birth. This was the explanation handed down to me and others in our family over the years, and with each retelling the circuits in the brain that made this seem plausible strengthened. But now, I'd decided, this explanation had a wobbly base indeed. To begin with, it seemed unlikely that an injury that severe could have occurred in the hospital without my parents knowing more. At the very least, a severe head injury would have prompted a call to a neurologist or neurosurgeon to evaluate and possibly treat a suspected hemorrhage in the brain. And the cover-up needed to conceal such a horrific accident would be something out of a medical thriller and not real life. To top it off, my parents weren't even sure what they'd been told, or by whom. It was pretty clear, I concluded, that my brother had not suffered a serious postnatal traumatic brain injury.

Next, I set out to collect the medical records, studies, and consultations related to my brother's medical history. These were pre-internet days, so the search required snail mail and legwork. I visited Flushing Hospital during spring break, and with consent forms and approvals from the medical staff, reviewed additional documents that might have revealed more about my brother's condition during the critical first few minutes of his life and the hours that followed. Could I uncover something that others had missed? I walked the floor of the neonatal unit hoping to find someone who could remember the terribly sick Hauser baby, but it was now more than 15 years since Howard's birth, 7 since his death, and my search for eyewitnesses proved futile. I spoke with our family doctor who had cared for Howard after he left the hospital and reviewed the note from the well-known consultant neurologist who examined my brother in his Manhattan office.

The hospital records were useless; they might as well have been written by healthcare aides, not medical professionals. Just a few words—"Poor color, not responding, not feeding"—plus charts of temperature, pulse, blood pressure, height, weight, that sort of thing. But not a word about a possible cause or what had happened. No mention of a fall. No studies or investigations. No diagnosis. No note about the frightened, frantic, tearful mom.

The consultant neurologist wasn't much better. His note was also just a single line: "severe mental and physical retardation, likely prenatal asphyxia" (loss of oxygen to the brain). My parents had been told that he knew more about mental retardation than anyone else in the entire city, and my mom, on a mission, had fought to secure an appointment, for which she had to pay a week's salary up front. They hoped he'd be able to suggest something so that one day Howard might be able to walk or talk. As Mom later told me, when the day arrived, my folks bundled up their two-year-old child and headed to the doctor's swank office on Manhattan's East Side. After a brief exam, he told them curtly that there was no hope and hustled them out the door. The whole thing had lasted ten minutes, max.

Mom was devastated. It wasn't just the prognosis—she suspected this—but the ice-cold way that the news was conveyed signaled that she and my dad were alone. The medical community, unable to fix Howard's problem, had washed its hands of him, and them.

The neurologist's diagnosis was probably correct, but his care was abysmal. Was there no time in his schedule for kindness? If he'd been just a little bit nicer, even if he couldn't do anything for Howard, he'd have helped so much more.

I never discovered with certainty what happened to my brother, but at least I could formulate a diagnosis with reasonably high confidence. Howard had extensive damage to both cerebral hemispheres, more or less equally, and especially to the posterior frontal and parietal-temporal lobes, a pattern of damage suggesting loss of blood supply from two major vessels in the brain, the paired middle cerebral arteries. His occipital lobes for vision and brain stem for eye movements and hearing were spared because these areas are nourished by other, more resilient arteries. A loss of oxygen or blood supply to the brain sometime late in gestation, or even at birth, was by far the most likely explanation for this pattern. This is a common cause of disability in children. It's similar to what happens following a cardiac arrest or suffocation—in medical terminology a hypoxic-ischemic encephalopathy—or after a stroke from blood clots in brain arteries. Had it happened earlier in pregnancy it would have left telltale signs—a small head, other abnormal features—none of which Howard had. Sometimes an infection is the culprit, but Mom had been healthy throughout the pregnancy, and there were no stigmata of infection. Genetic testing was not performed, but I'd learned enough about genetic causes of retardation to exclude a hereditary cause. Howard's high fevers were also a false lead; I was certain that these were not due to a misbehaving immune system but rather to damaged brain reflexes that failed to properly control my brother's swallowing, causing repeated aspiration of food into his lungs and recurrent pneumonias.

I reported back to my parents. "Mom and Dad, I'm pretty sure that Howard had terrible brain damage before he was born. This was probably caused by inadequate blood supply to the brain, like what happens with a stroke. We don't really know why this happened to him, or to many other children with a similar problem. The medical records show that Howard was very sick from the moment that he was born. This tells us that something happened before or during birth, and probably not after he was born. So I don't think that he was dropped."

Mom asked, "Why did he have such high fevers?"

"His swallowing reflexes were not working properly, and food sometimes went into his lungs, causing pneumonias."

I'd seen Mom cry before, many times, but never had I seen Dad's eyes well up with tears.

"Any idea why this happened?" he asked.

"I don't, Dad, not really. Most of the time we can't find a cause. It's not a genetic problem, though, so I don't think that David or I need to worry about our kids in the future."

"Thank God," Mom whispered.

"I think that it was just bad luck," I said. "I also think that you did a wonderful, amazing job with Howard, and with us."

My dad then spoke. "This all makes sense to me."

I found no smoking gun, but was able to give my parents some relief, even if the tragedy of Howard's life would continue to haunt them for the rest of their lives.

And even though I wasn't able to uncover something conclusive about what had caused my brother's condition, I learned things about medicine that would direct my path moving forward. A particularly important insight came from the greatest neurologist at Harvard Medical School, Raymond D. Adams, head of the department. His classic textbook* had laid out a modern approach to neurologic diagnosis, becoming a bible for clinicians around the world, and he'd also codified the causes of mental retardation and the approach to solving enigmatic cases. Bob DeLong arranged for me to meet with him, in person, one-on-one.

Tall and bald, with a ramrod-straight athletic frame and a penetrating gaze, Adams was a man of few words and strong opinions, frankly expressed. An imposing figure to his peers, and a terrifying one to medical students. When I went up to his office, he asked me what I wanted to study. I said mental retardation.

"I don't think that you can fix that problem," Adams told me. "Better to work on something that you can solve."

* * *

Most of the students I knew at Harvard Medical School believed in service and wanted to accomplish big things. Money was less of a priority; for me, it was not even on my radar. Apart from tuition and board, which my parents had provided, I needed little. Pizza from Regina in a quiet corner of the North End, or Thai food on Charles Street so hot that your mouth would tingle for hours in the cold night air—these were the things I loved. And I didn't need much space, just a studio, or at most a one-bedroom apartment in the Back Bay or Fenway, neighborhoods that were still affordable then.

I've forgotten much of what I learned in medical school classrooms, but I remember virtually everything from the top-of-field physicians I observed who'd answer calls for help, often on weekends or at odd hours of the night, from people

---

* *Principles of Neurology*, Raymond D. Adams and Maurice Victor, McGraw Hill, 1977.

experiencing the worst moment of their lives. I'd trail them as they'd walk down to the emergency ward or climb stairs to the hospital floor, watching them minister to people they'd never met before; the best of them did so with skill, compassion, and patience. I'd also observe the bad examples—one in particular would approach every patient with a scowl. Famously arrogant, he was brusque and short with patients and colleagues alike. He was an excellent diagnostician, the guy you'd want for a hard case that nobody could put their finger on, but he was terrible at the caring part of medical care. And whenever he was around there was no joy in the work.

I learned how not to behave from him.

CHAPTER 15

The Bs and Ts

Albert Coons, who taught us immunology, was a tall, patrician figure who'd lecture in a monotone while pacing back and forth, frequently inhaling asthma medicine from a spray canister. Coons was renowned for developing a method to label immune molecules called antibodies with colored fluorescent tags so that their specific target could be identified. This discovery revolutionized the diagnosis of infectious and autoimmune disorders. For the first time it became possible looking under a microscope to visualize the exact virus or bacterium that was responsible for an infection, or to pinpoint a rogue antibody injuring a healthy cell in the body.

Coons was present at the birth of modern concepts of autoimmunity, the attack by a wayward immune system against healthy tissues of the body. Autoimmune disease can strike any organ: the bowels in ulcerative colitis, joints in rheumatoid arthritis, pancreas in diabetes mellitus, many different organs in lupus, and the brain in MS. Over a 40-year career as a physician-scientist, Coons had arrived at a new understanding of how these diseases might develop. Our immune system is an amazingly efficient fighting force, he'd say, fine-tuned by evolution, composed of 100 million unique units, each one able to respond to a different provocation. The system is capable of coordinated activity but also has wide berth to respond individually to local conditions on the ground. This diversity permits targeted warfare against, for example, a poliovirus infection, without also calling out the specialized units that evolved to battle flu, or the myriad of other organisms that live in and on our body. And another axiom is that in the process of fighting infection, a normal immune system should never harm the host. But in autoimmune disease this is exactly what happens, due to a failure early in life to remove bad-actor immune cells or an inability to constrain them later on.

I was hooked, and set out to learn as much as I could. My timing was good, because a new wave of advances in studying cells and genes was ready to transform the field of immunology, and there was an increasing recognition of the clinical importance of autoimmune diseases.

The immune system is made up of exquisite interlocking parts, and when the pieces fit together perfectly, the outcome is magisterial, a symphony. Orchestrating this symphony are the lymphocytes, small white blood cells that circulate in the bloodstream and travel throughout the body. Lymphocytes come in two main types, T cells and B cells. T cells, by far the most abundant, are named for the thymus gland behind the chest wall where they are born. B cells are named for the bursa of Fabricius, an organ in chickens where the cells were first identified. Humans don't have a bursa, and at the time we didn't yet know that our B cells are produced in the bone marrow. T cells and B cells are "educated" in early life to attack invaders, such as infections, while not harming healthy tissues of the body.

B cells produce highly specific chemical bullets called antibodies. Each B cell is individually able to manufacture a unique antibody that recognizes only one adversary, usually a small structure of a particular shape and electrical charge. Antibodies are made up of four proteins that fit and fuse together to form a molecule with unique front and back ends. The front end binds to the specific substance recognized—its target—such as a protein from an infecting organism. There are millions of different possible front ends. Once the front end is bound, the back end either activates a cascade of proteins called "complement," or sticks to another type of lymphocyte appropriately called a "killer cell." In either case, the target is pulverized.

At the time, not much was known about B cells (they'd only been discovered five years earlier), but there was one intriguing, and surprising, finding. In mice born without B cells, T cells were also abnormal; they failed to function properly. This indicated that B and T cells don't act in isolation but rather communicate extensively with one another. We now know that when they recognize similar substances, they send messages in the form of chemicals to each other and to other cells in the vicinity, instructing them to turn on or off. Only a few chemical signals that coordinate B cell interactions with other immune cells had been identified back then,* but many others have since been found.

An even more consequential role for B cells would later be discovered. B cells are highly efficient antigen-presenting cells, meaning they can partner with T cells that respond to the same substance as the B cells and, depending on the situation, activate or inactivate T cells in the vicinity. And working synergistically, B and T cells together produce substances that can regulate a host of other immune cells, not only lymphocytes but also macrophages, monocytes, brain microglia, and others. Why is this important? Because it explains how small numbers of B cells could control the activity of the entire immune system. It would take nearly half a century before this process was recognized as the key to understanding MS.

We also didn't know back then that bacteria and viruses need

---

* Interleukin-4 (IL-4) was the first mediator identified that stimulated B cells.

to be around for B and T cells to work properly. Some bugs cool down the messaging, while others heat it up, and the immune system evolved to work in their presence. Laboratory animals raised in germ-free environments—think parents who constantly sanitize their kids' hands—have feeble immune systems; they are unable to fend off infections. They are also protected against developing autoimmune disease, but when infectious agents are introduced at a later age, aggressive immune diseases can appear.

Why should this be the case? As B and T cells respond to infections, cells that also react ("cross-react") with healthy tissues of the body should be removed. After all, eliminating these "autoreactive" cells is a big reason why B and T cells require education. But education is most effective early in life, so when bugs are first encountered in older individuals, school is out, and the autoreactive cells are no longer efficiently removed. Fortunately for us, even after we've reached maturity, some autoreactive cells that escape elimination can still be continuously suppressed or inactivated throughout life.

Lymphocytes that mistakenly attack healthy tissues are probably not eliminated as effectively as they were in our ancestors because fewer or different bugs are now encountered in early life. Our immune repertoire has been recast because we've disrupted the microbial world around us. And the result appears to be an epidemic of immune diseases in the developed world.

This revelation hit home. My asthma always worsened whenever I had the flu or a cold, so I knew that a close relationship must exist between infections and the level of inflammation in my lungs. It made sense that the immune system could be gated or regulated by viruses and bacteria in the environment. I now understood how my mononucleosis was almost certainly caused by a later-than-nature-intended encounter with the Epstein-Barr virus. And my search for immune causes of Howard's unexplained high fevers further piqued my interest in understanding the workings of our body's defense system. Seeds were planted that would blossom when I encountered the enigma of MS.

CHAPTER 16

Another Lesson in Neurology

By the time medical school came to a close, I was determined to become a neurologist. Nothing in medicine seemed more important than the brain, this three-pound organ, shaped like paired fists, the seat of intelligence and behavior, central command for all bodily functions. But the immune system seemed almost as enticing, and in a practical sense was more knowable than the brain: the field was exploding because immune cells could be studied from a simple tube of blood. As an immunologist, the opportunity to make real progress against brain disease seemed realistic. I didn't yet have a clear plan, but the pieces were beginning to come together.

After eight years away I was now back in New York, at New York Hospital on the east side of Manhattan, a resident in internal medicine. It was good to be close to home again, but all was not right. Grandpa Barney, Mom's dad, was unwell—his voice had softened, his gait had slowed, and his left hand was shaking. It was obvious that he had Parkinson's disease, but Grandpa refused to discuss it with any of us, not even his grandson, the budding neurologist. When asked how he felt, he'd say, "Nonsense; I'm fine."

Parkinson's disease is caused by the death of nerve cells that use the chemical dopamine to transmit information to other cells. Only 1 in 200 neurons in the brain make dopamine, but without these cells, movements are incapacitated.

It was long known that a chemical called L-dopa is converted to dopamine in the body, so maybe it could be used as a medicine to replace the dopamine from the cells that had died. A logical idea, but when tried, it didn't work. Until a stubborn Greek neurologist named George Cotzias entered the scene and began testing higher and higher doses, though still without benefit. But rather than giving up, he increased the dose even more, and, finally, at unheard of doses as high as 16 grams each day, it worked! And the rest was history—millions of lives would be helped. Cotzias accomplished this feat in 1967. It would be the last effective new treatment for a neurodegenerative disease until our MS therapy was FDA approved 50 years later.

L-dopa often works spectacularly well at the beginning, but as Parkinson's worsens, its benefits usually wear off and side effects, such as unwanted movements, become increasingly evident. This is what was happening to my grandfather. The stiffness that had initially loosened up with L-dopa had returned, and violent shaking in his hand was a source of embarrassment to him. So, he kept his fisted hand jammed tight in his pocket, shaking through the cloth. Perhaps a change in my grandfather's drug regimen would provide more effective control of his tremors, I thought, so I arranged for him to see Dr. Cotzias himself, who had moved to New York and was now one of my professors.

Dr. Cotzias and his team treated my grandfather like a VIP, providing superb care even though they could do little to improve the shaking. And, quietly, Grandpa continued to rely on the young doctors at the VA for prescriptions and care. He preferred the VA interns to our world-renowned Parkinson's experts. The VA was a more comfortable place for him, with its no-frills waiting room and other veterans around for company.

A few months later, I was paged with a message that my grandfather had been admitted to the cardiac care unit. He'd been short of breath for a couple days, and when he mentioned to Grandma that he had some chest pain that morning, she called Mom, who drove him to Manhattan and the ER of the hospital where his grandson worked.

It was my hospital. I was a medical resident on the service and believed I could guarantee that he'd receive red-carpet care. I helped arrange for the admission, and the intern responsible for his care was not only a superb physician but also a close friend.

It was sometime after midnight the next night when I received the nurse's call. Could I stop by to see my grandfather? He was confused, she said, and my presence might help orient him. He'd been fine when I spoke to him just a few hours earlier.

Despite my training, I was in no way prepared for the scene. As I entered the room, I heard Grandpa scream, "Get me out of here; I'm going home." Sweating profusely, he was tightly shackled to the bedrails with arm and leg restraints. Attempting to wrest himself free, he'd mostly wriggled out of the hospital gown, a threadbare, rear-tie monstrosity that barely covered anything under the best of conditions. Blood was oozing out of the puncture site where he'd pulled out his intravenous line, and he'd injured his urethra pulling out a catheter. The cardiac monitor wires, attached with sticky "leads" that painfully pulled off a thicket of chest hair each time that they were repositioned, were beeping chaotically on the EKG monitor overhead, a signal of cardiac disaster when the body is in repose but under these conditions a false alarm. Grandpa hadn't slept in this strange and unfriendly environment, where breathing machines, and intravenous drips, and drug monitors chirped without end, and where strangers entered every 30 minutes to check his pulse, blood pressure, and temperature, and just in case he might miraculously doze for a few minutes, they'd shine a flashlight in his eyes to check his pupils and shake him at the shoulders to ask if he was feeling any discomfort. Only the comatose sleep in the ICU.

To the hospital staff my grandfather was just another elderly man who'd "sundowned," meaning that he'd become confused and agitated in the evening. This is an everyday occurrence in hospitals that care for critically ill elderly people. The staff didn't know that my grandfather was a scholar, with interests in literature, history, and religion. They'd never seen him in the outside world, never witnessed his dignity, his formal dress no matter how hot it was outside, always a clean white shirt, often a tie, a traditional brimmed hat covering his bald head. All they saw was a screaming, incoherent elderly man.

When Grandpa saw me, he screamed again, "Get me out of here!" as the nurses gave him "something" to calm him down. It worked; as he became sedated, he stopped fighting the restraints, pulling on the tubes, and demanding to go home. Next morning, he was mostly back to his old self. Fortunately, he remembered little of the event, and the moment that our family returned in force, he signed out "against medical advice."

"Good riddance," he said, as the door closed behind him.

It would be the last time that my grandfather would ever agree to be hospitalized, and shortly after that horrible experience he told me he'd decided to stop the life-saving medicines to treat his Parkinson's disease. We both knew he needed those drugs to swallow his food and prevent choking. He asked me not to tell anyone else in the family. I think that the dehumanizing experience in my hospital, under the "very best possible" care by my colleagues and friends, hastened his decision to die on his own terms, dignity intact.

And he did, just a few days later.

The purpose of medicine is to treat the person, not the illness. The clinician must learn to see through the eyes of the patient.

CHAPTER 17

Experimenting on People

By 1977, I'd completed training in internal medicine and moved back to Boston to become a neurology resident at the Massachusetts General Hospital. The MGH was renowned for its neurology service and in particular for a remarkable trio of senior physicians, each of whom had made stellar contributions that had transformed the world's understanding of numerous brain diseases. Each would also play a decisive role in my education and career, providing a compass at critical junctures.

The first, Ray Adams, was the imposing head of the neurology department, who four years earlier had advised me not to work on mental retardation but instead find a problem that I could solve. The second, already introduced, was Charles Miller Fisher. And the third was Edward Pearson Richardson, a great figure in neuropathology who'd play a large role in my later work on MS.

Working with Dr. Fisher was a unique experience. A Canadian, he was one of the first soldiers captured by the Germans during World War II, and he remained a prisoner for six years. The main occupational risk of prison, he'd say, was boredom. But through good fortune, he was given responsibility for maintaining the officers' library, where he could spend the days immersed in books. He'd tell us that this experience taught him to never rush. Medicine was a quiet, contemplative profession in those days, but Dr. Fisher seemed to take it to extremes. He dug deep, and most everything attracted his curiosity.

Fisher rounds, our daily visits with his patients in the hospital, could last eight hours or more, but the time flew by. He taught us to observe, unhurriedly, and to write daily notes in no more than a line or two, "so as not to waste paper," he'd say, but really to force us to focus on what was truly important in the patient's care. He knew everyone's name and took an interest in our lives.

Fisher was tall, bald, and pale. He wore spanking white shirts, frayed at the cuffs, and a long, white, starched coat. Mr. Clean, but with black accents: eyebrows, thick glasses, and cavalry-shine shoes. He spoke softly, barely above a whisper, and with each curious or unexpected happening, he'd flash a bemused smile. He may have been the kindest person I've ever met. His patients worshipped him, and so did we.

Undiagnosed puzzles were his specialty. He'd approach each one slowly, deliberately, noninvasively, turning it over in his head until an answer emerged. He'd nurture new ideas at the bedside and validate them through meticulous study of brain pathology. His office was filled, ceiling to floor, with boxes containing thin slides of brain tissue, hundreds each from scores of patients whose postmortem specimens might provide a window into the cause of their illnesses during life. His desk was buried underneath the avalanche of slides and medical records, and visitors had to carefully navigate a narrow path he'd cleared so as not to topple the precious goods.

I once asked him what interested him the most, what was his greatest passion?

"The neurology of ungrateful," he replied.

He'd roam the hospital corridors late at night asking the nurses, the residents, anyone if they knew of any ungrateful, angry, irritated patients. In the days before strict rules for medical privacy were the norm, he'd enter the rooms of selected patients, armed with pen and notepad and smile, and cheerfully discuss with them the source of their unhappiness, separating out cases in which the ungrateful feeling was justified from those whose ungratefulness was caused by a brain problem. He'd carefully record these interviews and then wait, sometimes decades, for opportunities to examine the brains of these patients, hoping to find out where these behaviors lived in the brain.

One day I read a preliminary study in the medical journal *Lancet*, a prestigious publication with an unfortunate name that dates from the era of bloodletting. It said that a normal hormone, vasopressin, delivered via a simple nasal spray, could be given to people with dementia to improve memory! This seemed incredible to me, and on rounds that evening, after visiting an older woman with Alzheimer's disease, I shared the results of the study with Dr. Fisher, and we discussed together a plan to replicate the findings to see if it was true.

"Dr. Fisher, this is great," I said. "I'll write a letter to the Human Studies Committee to ask for permission to do this."

"That would take much too long," he replied. "We'll just come back later tonight when everyone is sleeping and the nurses aren't around. We can tiptoe into the patient's room and spray it into her nose while she's asleep. Don't tell anyone. When we come back in the morning, we can see if there's any difference."

"Dr. Fisher, I don't know that I'm permitted to do this."

"Don't worry," he responded.

And when we returned the next day, our patient was no better.

This was the state of medical research in the 1970s. The newly minted guidelines for conduct, outlined in 1974 as the Belmont principles, were not yet universally adopted, even at the Massachusetts General Hospital. Most important was the requirement of informed consent, meaning that participants must fully understand the nature of the study, the risks and possible benefits to themselves and others, and voluntarily agree, freely and without coercion, to undergo the experimental procedure or treatment. Throughout much of the 20th century, informed consent was required for experiments with healthy volunteers, but not always for patients.

In the late 1960s, Harvard's Henry Beecher had written influential articles detailing examples of medical abuse by his colleagues. Some involved violations of the principle of equipoise,* such as testing the value of antibiotics by treating some infected patients with a placebo. Others were shocking examples of lousy judgment. Beecher described a woman injected with her dying daughter's cancer cells in an effort to develop an antiserum. Instead, it transferred the deadly tumor to the mother.

He pulled no punches, and he named names. Big names. After publication, one can only imagine the scene when he first stopped in for lunch at the faculty club. *On the Waterfront*, Harvard style. Beecher sensitized the world to the importance of ethics in experimental medicine, and by the time I arrived on the scene in the late 1970s, a modern system of oversight had just been put in place. It hadn't yet filtered up to all the gray hairs, but to up-and-comers like me, the new rules were already ingrained in our DNA. There would be no more undercover experiments conducted in the dark of night.

---

* Equipoise in research means that uncertainty exists about the relative value of the approaches being tested.

CHAPTER 18

Learning from Patients

The title of "resident" is a carryover from the 19th century when physicians in training actually lived in the hospital. We no longer did, but given the demands of our schedules, we may as well have. I'd begin the day at 6:30 a.m., visiting the patients on my service, then work all day and half the nights without a break, usually six days a week. This was a schedule that would crush all but the young, but the payoff came in an incredibly high learning curve.

One of the first things Dr. Fisher taught me was to write down the stories of each patient I saw; otherwise, he cautioned, "you'll lose them forever." So I did. Over one busy eight-week period I cared for patients with every known type of neurologic disease, and this experience became the source for my first book, *Case Series in Neurology*, a compilation of clinical vignettes. I lived, as did many of my fellow residents, in a high-rise complex across the street from the hospital, and despite the workload we still found time for fun, dinners, and parties together, early morning ski trips to Vermont, outings to the beaches on Cape Cod. Lifelong bonds often form out of immersive experiences, and this was certainly the case for us. But most important, by far, was the work. Neurology was my life.

It was around this time that Dr. Fisher introduced me to Andrea, the young woman battling a terribly aggressive form of

MS whose story opens this book. This was not accidental; he'd often invite residents to care for patients he thought might have special meaning for us.

Andrea tore at my heart, and MS stoked my interest. I began to read everything that I could about the disease. And then, a few weeks later, I met a second patient, a woman who would influence my thinking more than anyone I've ever cared for.

Emily was a vibrant, professional woman in her late thirties, and I'd been scheduled to see her in clinic. Tall and thin, with straight blonde hair, blue eyes, and a narrow face, she looked Scandinavian.

"Doctor, I've had MS for almost 20 years. My first symptoms came when I was in college, I believe in my freshman year. I developed blurry vision in one eye, I think it was on the left. I went to student health. They said they couldn't find much. Maybe I needed glasses and should see an optometrist. But within a few weeks, it got better, so I never went back."

"Did you have any other symptoms at that time?" I asked. "Any pain?"

"Yes, I remember that my eye ached."

"Did your vision recover?

"Yes. But after that episode, whenever I'd run on hot days, my left eye would become blurry again. It always got better, though, quickly, as soon as I stopped exercising. After a few years, it seemed to go away, and I was fine."

This pretty much sealed the deal. She had optic neuritis, the medical term for inflammation of the optic nerve, the biological wires that carry visual information from the back of the eye to the brain. An aching eye was typical in people with MS, and recurrent blurring with heat and exercise was a sure sign that the nerve was demyelinated—stripped of its protective insulation—and would short-circuit under stress.

Optic neuritis is a classic symptom of MS.

"Did you ever have any other symptoms?"

"Oh, yes," she replied, "I had several more attacks, maybe one, sometimes two, each year. I remember one with numbness in my leg. I don't remember which leg. Another time I had dizziness, and my walking was a little bit unsteady, and once I remember waking up and feeling numb from the waist down. But I recovered pretty well each time. In my senior year of college, student health sent me to a neurologist. He examined me and did a spinal tap. He then called me and said on the telephone that I had multiple sclerosis. Just like that. I had no idea what MS was. I asked him what that meant. He said that I'd have more attacks and probably would be in a wheelchair one day. There was no empathy in his voice. It was matter of fact."

"What did you do?"

"I asked him if there was any treatment. He said no, there was nothing that could be done. So, I hung up and decided not to see any more neurologists."

I'd heard similar stories often enough not to doubt that it really happened pretty much as she told it. "Then what happened?"

"It's interesting," she said. "The attacks stopped, and I just sort of forgot about it."

"Why did you come in today?" I asked.

"Well, Dr. Swan is my friend, and she suggested that I see you, just to make sure that I'm doing everything I should. I haven't seen a neurologist in more than ten years."

She looked entirely healthy, an appearance quickly confirmed by a neurological exam. I knew that benign MS existed, but I'd never seen anyone who'd had the disease for so long and yet seemed free of any impairment.

"Do you have any MS symptoms now?" I asked.

"Of course," she told me. "I never feel a hundred percent well."

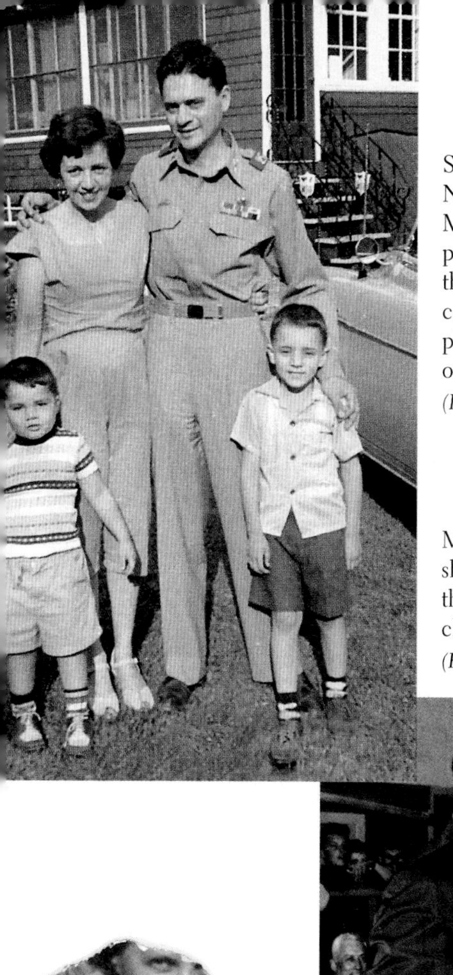

Summer at Olde Forge, New York, in the Adirondack Mountains in the 1950s, with my parents and brother David (on the left). The many trips to the countryside, prescribed by local physicians to help my asthma, only seemed to make it worse. *(Personal collection)*

Mom's brother, my Uncle Sandy, shown on the right, playing to the crowd with legendary boxing champion Jack Dempsey. *(Photo courtesy of Sanford Redock)*

My brother Howard, age 6 months, held by me, and both of us cradled by Grandma Rose. Howard would never be able to walk, understand language, or care for himself. When he died, Mom destroyed all of the photos she could find; this torn remnant is one of the few surviving images. *(Personal collection)*

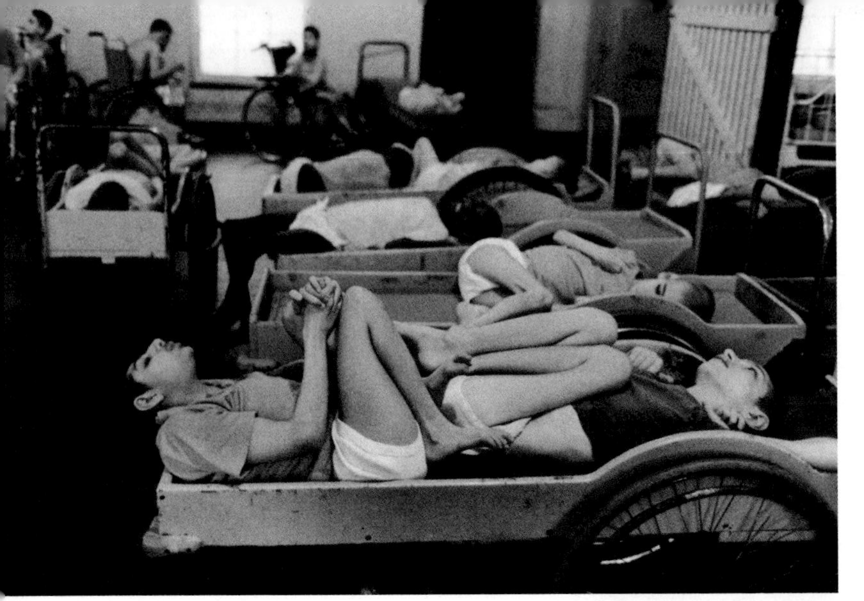

The Willowbrook State School in Staten Island, circa 1972, was typical of the era's public institutions for the physically and mentally disabled. My parents were determined to care for my brother Howard at home for as long as possible.
(Photo reprinted from Bill Pierce/The LIFE Images Collection/Getty)

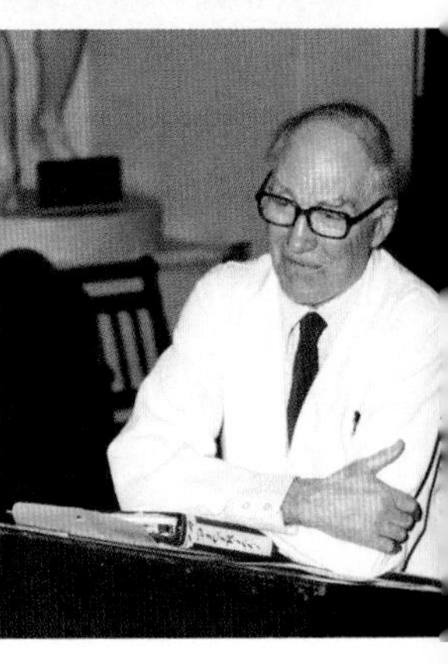

Raymond Adams was the greatest neurologist of his era. This 1970s photo was taken at the Ether Dome auditorium at the Massachusetts General Hospital. *(Photo courtesy of Robert Laureno, MD)*

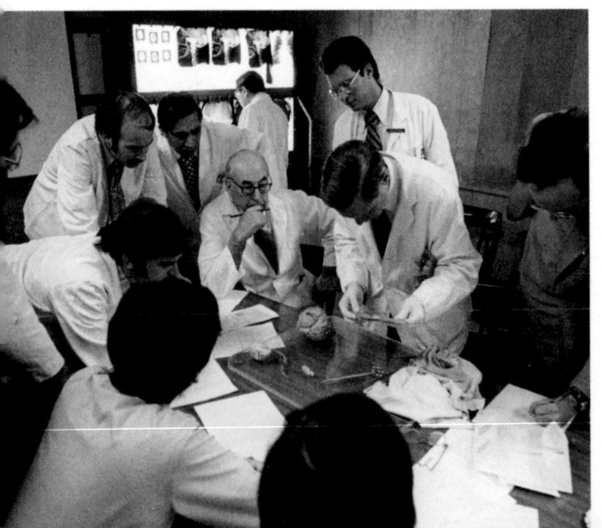

In the era before modern brain imaging, weekly brain-cutting sessions were the bes way to understand the cause of a patient's demise. Here, a seated Charles Miller Fisher pencil in hand, is gazing at the undersurface of a recentl removed brain. Standing and partially bent over in the foreground is E. P. Richardso the great neuropathologist at Harvard.
(Photo courtesy of Allan H. Ropp MD, standing just behind Fisher

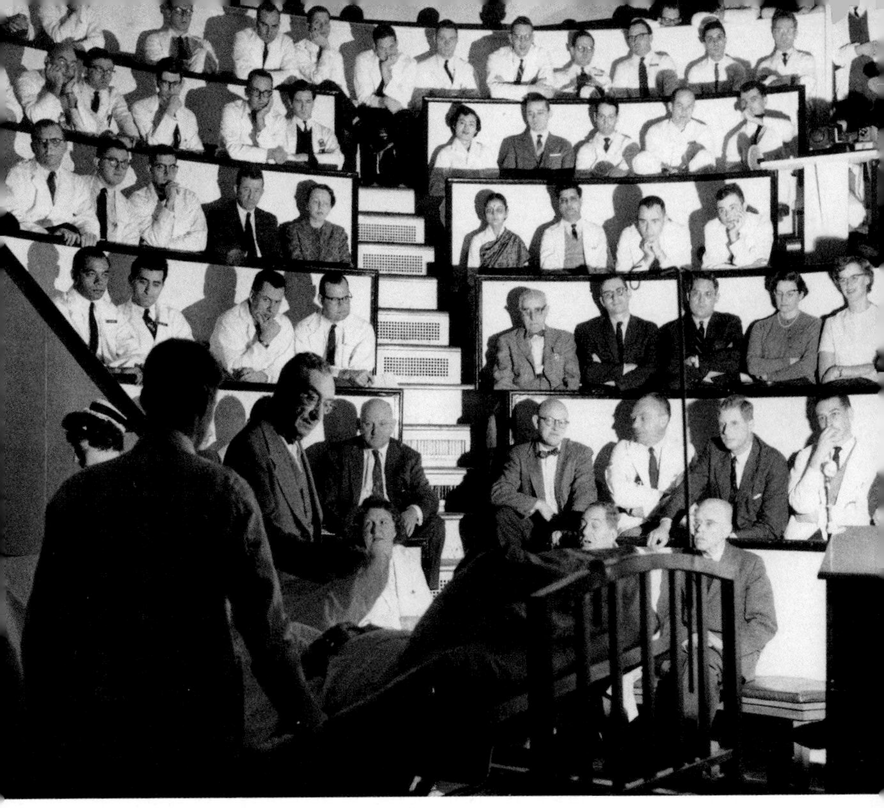

The Ether Dome at the Massachusetts General Hospital was a small, formal amphitheater with rapidly ascending rows of wooden seats packed together. The atmosphere was intense and could be daunting for trainees.

(Massachusetts General Hospital Archives, with permission)

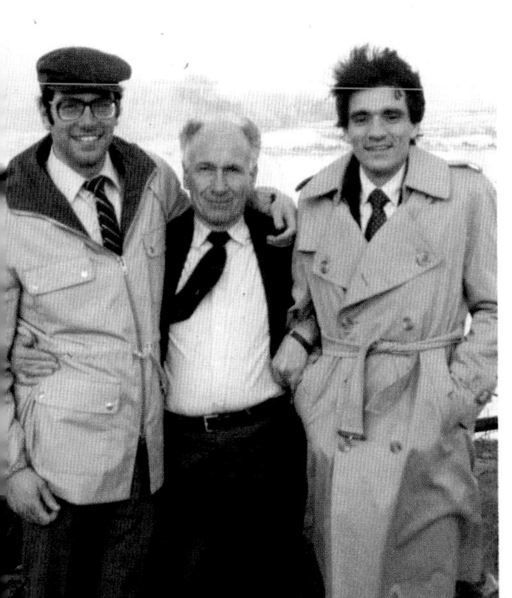

With my colleagues Howard Weiner (left) and the immunologist Byron Waksman (center) of the National Multiple Sclerosis Society at an excursion to nearby Niagara Falls during the MS Society's 1982 meeting at Grand Island, New York, where the results of our cyclophosphamide trial in MS were first presented.

(Photo courtesy of Howard L. Weiner, MD)

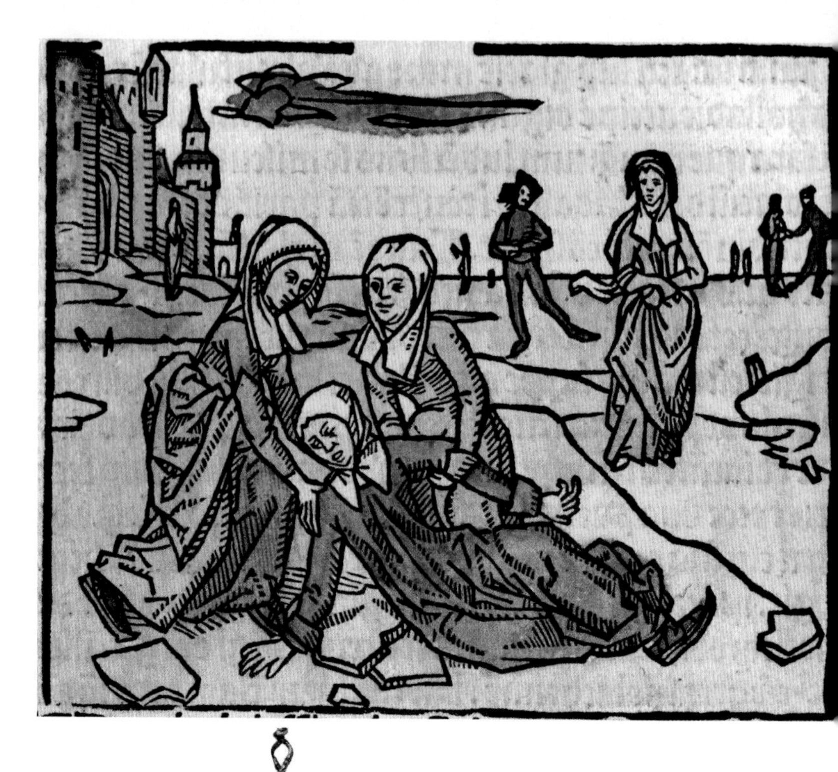

The cloudy historical trail of autoimmune disease. Above: a 15th-century image of Lidwina (1380–1433), a mystic and saint, and possibly a person with MS although accounts of her illness are too vague to be certain. *(Johannes Brugman, 1498)* Left: a childhood portrait of Augustus Frederick d'Este (1794–1848). The illegitimate grandson of King George III, Augustus is the first historical personage with a convincing history of MS, thanks to a detailed diary that he maintained throughout his life. *(Image by Richard Cosway: 1799, Victoria and Albert Museum)*

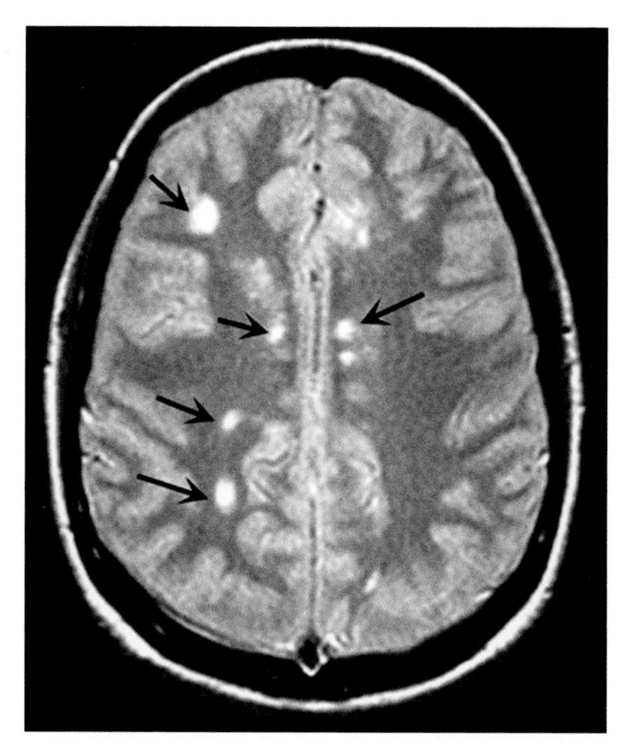

An MRI image from a patient with early MS. This horizontal view of the brain shows numerous white spots (arrows), indicating areas of demyelination and scarring. MRI has transformed the understanding of MS.
(Reproduced from Harrison's Principles of Internal Medicine, *21st Edition, 2022, with permission from McGraw Hill)*

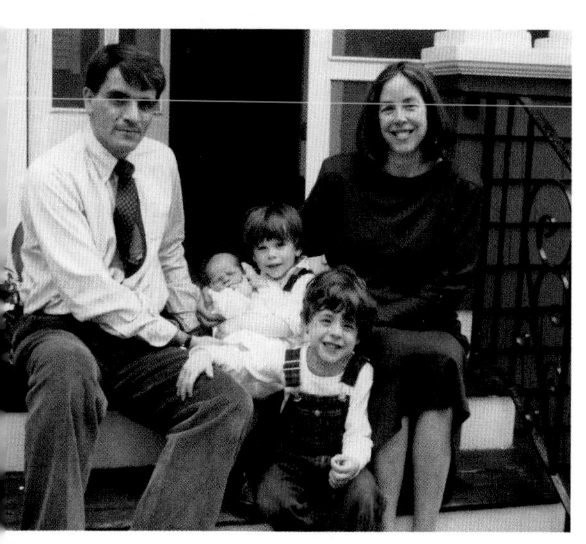

Returning to the US from Paris, we were a young family in an old town. Here, on the porch of our home in Concord, Massachusetts, a suburb of Boston, Elizabeth and I are introducing our two boys to their new baby brother.
(Personal collection)

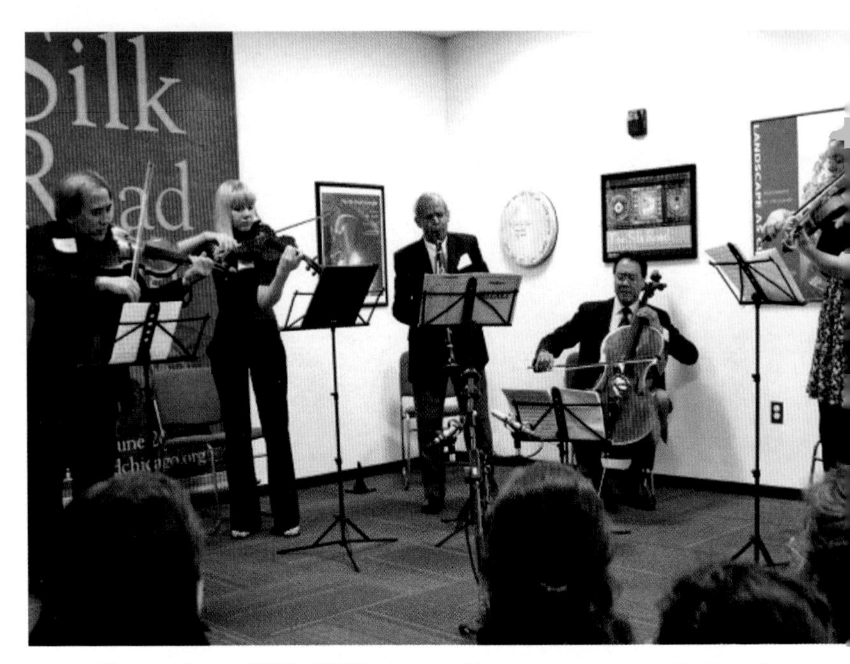

Norman Letvin (1949–2012) pioneered immune system investigations in nonhuman primates, making possible the development of an improved animal model for MS. He was also a brilliant musician. This photo shows him (standing, center) performing for the Silk Road Project at Harvard. Seated to Norman's left is cellist YoYo Ma. *(Photo courtesy of Marion Stein, MD)*

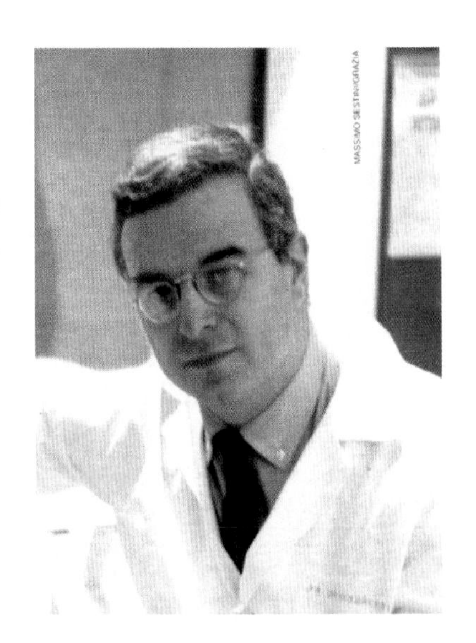

Luca Massacesi, now professor of neurology in Florence, Italy. As a postdoctoral fellow, Luca figured out the recipe needed to create an MS-like disease in Callithrix marmosets. This was the first breakthrough.
(Photo courtesy of Luca Massacesi)

Neurologist Craig Smith at Genentech was a powerful advocate for testing the high-risk strategy of B cell therapy for MS and helped lead the rituximab trial; he is also a national champion rower. *(Photo courtesy of Craig Smith)*

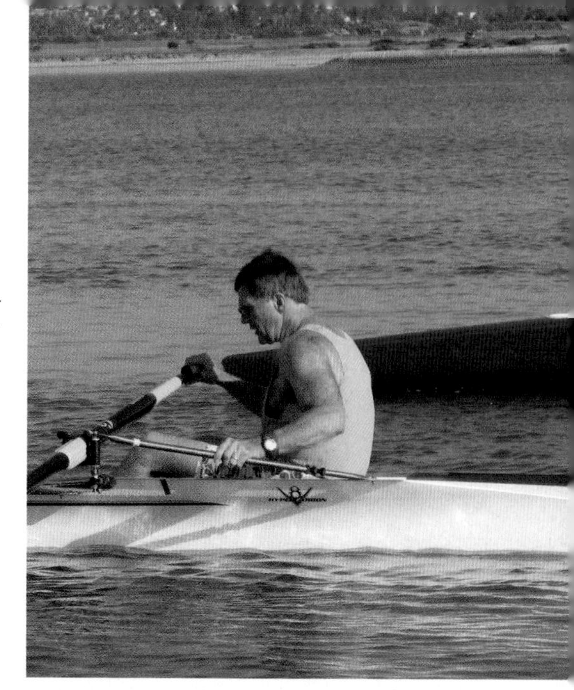

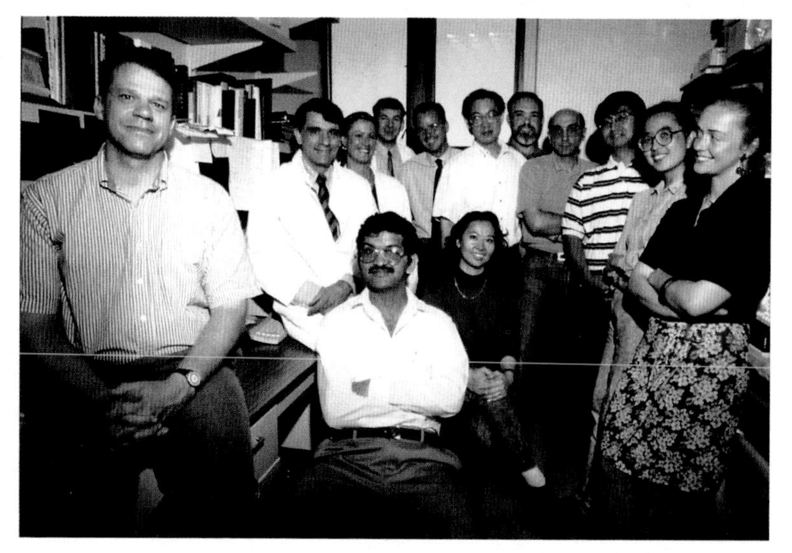

Our lab team in the 1990s. Claude Genain (left foreground, seated on desk) made the key discovery that antibodies and B cells produced MS-like lesions; I'm in a white coat, seated behind Claude; Jorge Oksenberg (bearded, rear) and Robin Lincoln (standing to my left) led the African American genetics program; Emmanuelle Waubant (far right) helped design the rituximab trial; and David Leppert (on Robin's left) would later play important roles at Roche/Genentech and Novartis in developing B cell therapeutics for MS. *(Photo courtesy of Robin Lincoln)*

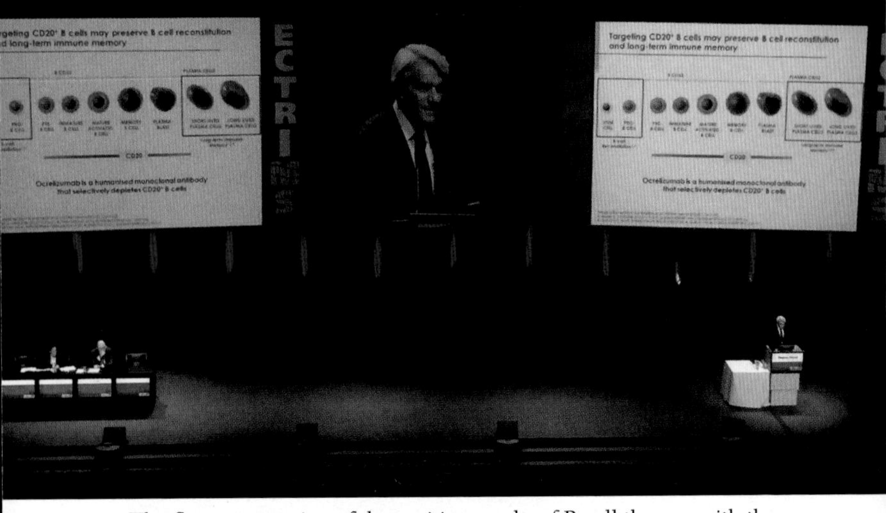

The first presentation of the exciting results of B cell therapy with the new drug ocrelizumab in patients with MS, and the culmination of a 40-year journey to understand and treat this common and disabling disease of the nervous system. Barcelona, Spain, October 2015. *(Personal collection)*

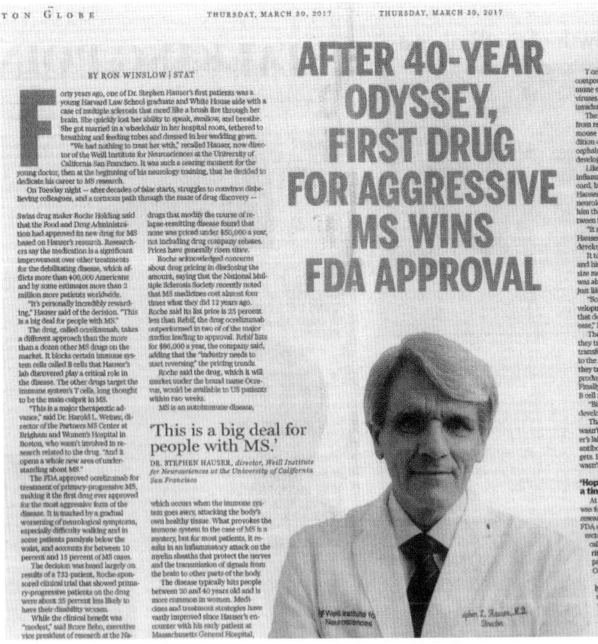

THE BOSTON GLOBE THURSDAY, MARCH 30, 2017

AFTER 40-YEAR ODYSSEY, FIRST DRUG FOR AGGRESSIVE MS WINS FDA APPROVAL

BY RON WINSLOW | STAT

Forty years ago, one of Dr. Stephen Hauser's first patients was a young Harvard Law School graduate and White House aide with a case of multiple sclerosis that raced like a brush fire through her brain. She quickly lost her ability to speak, swallow, and breathe. She got married in a wheelchair in her hospital room, tethered to breathing and feeding tubes and dressed in her wedding gown.

"We had nothing to treat her with," recalled Hauser, now director of the Weill Institute for Neurosciences at the University of California San Francisco. It was such a searing moment for the young doctor, then at the beginning of his neurology training, that he decided to dedicate his career to MS research.

On Tuesday night — after decades of false starts, struggles to convince disbelieving colleagues, and a tortuous path through the maze of drug discovery — Swiss drug maker Roche Holding said that the Food and Drug Administration had approved its new drug for MS based on Hauser's research. Researchers say the medication is a significant improvement over other treatments for the debilitating disease, which afflicts more than 400,000 Americans and by some estimates more than 2 million more patients worldwide.

"It's personally incredibly rewarding," Hauser said of the decision. "This is a big deal for people with MS."

The drug, called ocrelizumab, takes a different approach than the more than a dozen other MS drugs on the market. It blocks certain immune system cells called B cells that Hauser's lab discovered play a critical role in the disease. The other drugs target the immune system's T cells, long thought to be the main culprit in MS.

"This is a major therapeutic advance," said Dr. Harold L. Weiner, director of the Partners MS Center at Brigham and Women's Hospital in Boston, who wasn't involved in research related to the drug. "And it opens a whole new area of understanding about MS."

The FDA approved ocrelizumab for treatment of primary-progressive MS, making it the first drug ever approved for the most aggressive form of the disease. It is marked by a gradual worsening of neurological symptoms, especially difficulty walking and in some patients paralysis below the waist, and accounts for between 10 percent and 15 percent of MS cases.

The decision was based largely on results of a 732-patient, Roche-sponsored clinical trial that showed primary-progressive patients on the drug were about 25 percent less likely to have their disability worsen.

While the clinical benefit was "modest," said Bruce Bebo, executive vice president of research at the Na- drugs that modify the course of relapse-remitting disease found that none was priced under $50,000 a year, not including drug company rebates. Prices have generally risen since.

Roche acknowledged concerns about drug pricing in disclosing the amount, saying that the National Multiple Sclerosis Society recently noted that MS medicines cost almost four times what they did 12 years ago. Roche said its list price is 25 percent less than Rebif, the drug ocrelizumab outperformed in two of of the major studies leading to approval. Rebif lists for $86,000 a year, the company said, adding that the "industry needs to start reversing" the pricing trends.

Roche said the drug, which it will market under the brand name Ocrevus, would be available to US patients within two weeks.

MS is an autoimmune disease,

> 'This is a big deal for people with MS.'
>
> DR. STEPHEN HAUSER, *director, Weill Institute for Neurosciences at the University of California San Francisco*

which occurs when the immune system goes awry, attacking the body's own healthy tissue. What provokes the immune system in the case of MS is a mystery, but for most patients, it results in an inflammatory attack on the myelin sheaths that protect the nerves and the transmission of signals from the brain to other parts of the body.

The disease typically hits people between 20 and 40 years old and is more common in women. Medicines and treatment strategies have vastly improved since Hauser's encounter with his early patient at Massachusetts General Hospital,

T cells, as well as B cells, are key components of the arsenal the immune system uses to detect and kill viruses, bacteria, and other "foreign" invaders that harm the body.

The focus on T cells grew in part from researchers' longtime use of a mouse model with a T cell-driven condition called experimental allergic encephalomyelitis, or EAE, to study and develop drugs for the disease.

Like MS, EAE is characterized by inflammation of the brain and spinal cord, but there, the similarities end. Hauser's mentor, the late Harvard neurologist Dr. Raymond Adams, told him there was little resemblance between the two conditions.

"It really didn't look like MS at all," Hauser said. So his first task was to develop a new animal model.

It took a decade, but eventually he and his lab came up with a guinea pig-size monkey called a marmoset that was able to develop MS that looked just like the human version.

"So many of our failures in drug development relate to preclinical models that don't recapitulate human disease," Hauser said.

Then, in a series of experiments, they tried to induce the disease by transferring myelin-targeted T cells into the animals. It didn't work. Next, they tried certain antibodies that are produced by B cells. That didn't work. Finally, they used both T cells and the B cell antibodies together.

"Bingo," Hauser said. The animals developed MS.

The experiments showed that MS wasn't fueled just by T cells, and Hauser's lab identified B cells and related antibodies as promising new drug targets. But the scientific establishment wasn't ready to embrace this new idea.

'Hoping to see a tiny whiff of effect'

At first, it seemed Hauser's timing was fortuitous. In 1997, as his group's research was coming together, the FDA approved the first treatment directed against B cells. It was a genetically engineered antibody called rituximab, from Genentech and its partner Idec Pharmaceuticals Corp.

The drug was for non-Hodgkin lymphoma, but its approval meant an off-the-shelf therapy was available to test their B cell hypothesis in MS patients.

Armed with journal articles describing their research, Haus-

ing MS on placebo for a year. Instead, the agency permitted only a single dose of the drug. The researchers would have to measure its effectiveness after just 24 weeks. Their hopes for success dimmed.

The study enrolled 104 patients, 6[…] of whom were treated with rituxima[…] The moment of truth came on what Hauser recalled was a crisp Friday af[…]ternoon in late September 2006 whe[…] the researchers "unblinded" the data. What they saw astonished them.

The formation of new brain lesio[…] in the rituximab patients was reduce[…] by 91 percent compared with those o[…] placebo. The size of the effect was "u[…]precedented" in MS, Hauser said. Th[…] study showed not only that B cells were critical players in the disease, b[…] that when B cells were depleted by th[…] drug, brain inflammation was almos[…] immediately shut down.

Said Hauser: "It was a grand slam home run."

It would take a much larger Phas[…] 3 trial to win FDA approval, but he fi[…]ured rituximab would be available to MS patients within four years — by about 2010.

Genentech 'had a better molecule'

Genentech had other ideas. Ritu[…]imab was an aging medicine, and it had safety issues. The company thought it had a better molecule, called ocrelizumab, to work with.

Hauser agreed that ocrelizumab would likely prove a better drug. Bu[…] he believed it would further delay g[…]ting a B cell therapy to patients.

The Phase 3 studies that led to F[…] approval were launched in 2011.

The results, which for the studie[…] relapsing patients were a near-repli[…]tion of the "grand slam" rituximab findings from 2006, were published the New England Journal of Medic[…] in December.

The two Roche-funded studies i[…]volving a total of 1,656 patients wit[…] relapsing MS showed the drug cut [...]nualized relapse rates for such patients almost in half compared with commonly used treatment called R[…]bif. The formation of new lesions i[…] the brain and spinal cord — the key marker of inflammation — was reduced by more than 94 percent co[…]pared to patients on Rebif. Why the [re]duction in relapse rates wasn't eve[…] more pronounced isn't clear.

"We've never had a treatment s[…] successful against new lesions," sa[…]

At long last, the first B cell therapy for MS receives FDA approval. (Boston Globe, *March 30, 2017; Ron Winslow for STAT News*)

She had chronic fatigue, brain fog from time to time, and she'd notice numbness in her legs whenever her body temperature rose, from heat, exercise, or an illness with fever. Also, when she bent her neck, a tingling sensation would shoot down her back and into her legs. All of these symptoms were typical for MS and left little doubt that the diagnosis was correct. But why was she doing so well, and were there lessons here for other, far less fortunate patients?

I asked about other illnesses. She was a cancer survivor. At age 24, just after graduating from business school, she developed breast cancer that had spread to her lymph nodes. It required intensive treatment with chemotherapy, including a particularly toxic drug called cyclophosphamide, known by its trade name Cytoxan. And then she told me something amazing.

"You know, Doctor, after the breast cancer, my MS attacks seemed to stop. In fact, for the past decade, they've pretty much gone away."

I wondered, could the chemotherapy have turned off her MS? Is this the reason why her MS had been so benign? Cyclophosphamide, the drug used in many chemotherapy regimens, disrupts the genetic machinery of dividing cells by chemically changing DNA, the building blocks of life.* Cancer cells divide rapidly, and this is why many cancers are sensitive to the drug. The same is true for infection-fighting white blood cells, contributing to the well-known risk for infection from chemotherapy.

Maybe killing lymphocytes could help people with MS.

This concept was certainly not novel. Lymphocytes had long been known to flood into brain tissue in patients with MS. However, the prevailing view was that MS must be caused by

---

* More specifically, cyclophosphamide acts as an alkylating agent that binds and chemically alters guanine, one of the four building blocks of DNA.

infection with a virus. If true, then suppressing the immune system would weaken host defenses and worsen the infection. MS would worsen. But contrary to expectations, immune suppression seemed to help Emily's MS. I began to wonder if my patient's story, this single experiment of nature, challenged a central maxim in the field. Were the lymphocytes themselves the culprit?

* * *

Emily's experience led me to consider the possibility of launching a clinical trial of immune suppression in people with MS. And word began to spread that I had a special interest in neuroimmune diseases. I began working off-hours in an immunology lab, and found to my enormous satisfaction that other physicians were sending patients my way and asking for my opinion. I was still a trainee, so this type of validation was extremely gratifying.

I was on a mission, absorbing everything I could about different ways to modulate immunity and how immune therapies affected people with autoimmune diseases of all types. I sought out patients with these conditions, and closely followed their progress. I began to road test new ideas at the bedside, and whenever possible in the lab. Then another memorable patient came into my world.

Rosella, a woman in her early forties, suffered from two unrelated problems: sarcoidosis and MS. Sarcoidosis is an immune disorder caused by rogue white blood cells that inflame lung tissue and sometimes other organs. Like MS, it's a chronic condition featuring episodic attacks and periods of remission. When sarcoidosis is active, it turns off the immune system, suppressing the activity of lymphocytes and leading to a heightened risk for infections.

As Rosella began to speak, I quickly realized the importance of her story. Here was confirmation of my theory. One patient is only an anecdote, but two become experience, a case series.

"It's really confusing to me," she said, "but maybe you can understand it. My MS seems to flare up whenever the sarcoidosis is in remission. When my sarcoidosis is active, the MS turns off. I either have one or the other, but never the two together."

Rosella's sarcoidosis experience immediately called to mind Emily's saga with cyclophosphamide. When the immune system is turned on, MS flares up. Suppress immunity, and MS goes into hibernation. I was beginning to feel confident that a story was developing to justify a study of immune suppression as treatment for MS.

MS treatment at the time, cynically summarized by a noted specialist, was "diagnose and adios."* Perhaps the cynicism was justified. Many MS patients had been subjected to ineffective and sometimes dangerous treatments without any real evidence that they might be effective. But amid a mountain of hokum, a few sober voices were beginning to suggest that rational treatment might be possible.

I zeroed in on two published papers, the first in 1975 by Otto Hommes, a Dutch neurologist in Nijmegen, and a second two years later by Richard Gonsette, a Belgian neurosurgeon. Both had treated people with aggressive MS using cyclophosphamide, and both reported that the treatment had stabilized the disease for periods of two years or longer.

These studies had many problems. They were uncontrolled, meaning that there was no untreated group used for comparison, and everyone—patients and investigators alike—knew that they'd been treated with the drug. This meant that a

* Labe Scheinberg, who worked at the Albert Einstein College of Medicine in New York.

placebo effect was possible. Also, it was not clear exactly what types of MS patients had been treated in these studies. Though the different categories of MS had not yet been systematically delineated—this would not occur until "official" diagnostic criteria were first proposed in 1983—we knew that some patients had relapsing forms of MS that could stabilize naturally over time, while others had progressive forms that almost always continued to steadily worsen. More clinical information, and a control group, would be needed to really determine if cyclophosphamide had any benefits on MS.

In spite of these reservations, I thought that the 141 patients treated by Hommes and the 83 by Gonsette may have revealed something profound about MS, perhaps a treatment that could be used immediately to help people with severe disease. I wrote to both and was beyond delighted when they responded positively and shared, first by mail and then by phone, details of their experience with cyclophosphamide and suggestions for how I might begin a study.* I then spoke with Ray Adams, and he suggested that I prepare a department-wide seminar to introduce my patients, describe the cyclophosphamide studies, review the history of attempts to treat MS, and present my embryonic plan.

---

* Otto Hommes was particularly encouraging. We arranged to meet at an upcoming neurology conference in the United States, but he was denied entry because of prior trips to North Vietnam, where he taught medicine and promoted healthcare, and because of his refusal to sign a loyalty oath as prerequisite for a visa. I was disappointed, angry, and ashamed that he was not allowed to attend.

CHAPTER 19

The Rehearsal

In preparation for the upcoming seminar, the first item of business was to undertake a comprehensive review of the literature. I was still in training, and was determined not to miss any information that could reveal an embarrassing lack of depth or, far worse, lead me to propose a clinical study that might harm rather than help patients. So I did my best to cover all cutting-edge research in the field. I also knew that I'd be facing strong headwinds from my colleagues. Neurology at the time was a cautious, conservative specialty. Other specialists would sometimes snicker that "neurologists know everything and do nothing." I was warned that "the surest way to ruin one's career is to propose a treatment for MS."* These considerations only strengthened my resolve to leave no stone unturned as I formulated the strongest possible case for my clinical study.

In the late 1970s, new findings in biomedical research were communicated slowly. There was no internet, no e-anything, not even fax machines. We'd typically wait weeks or months to receive medical articles printed in journals.

That meant a trip to the basement of Harvard's Countway Medical Library to read through the annual *Cumulated Index*

---

* Attributed to Houston Merritt, chief of neurology at Columbia and co-discoverer of phenytoin (Dilantin) as treatment for epilepsy.

Medicus, the huge, hardbound series of volumes listing all papers published on all subjects in medicine during the previous years. Papers published in the current year were listed in softcover monthly issues. There was a delay of several months between the publication of an article and its listing in the *Index Medicus*, so to ensure I was up to date, I manually scanned recent issues of all individual journals likely to publish articles in my area.

Knowing the location of every copy machine in the library was an essential part of a researcher's skill set. At each machine, there was typically a line, three or four deep, of harried researchers waiting their turn, pockets bulging with the nickels, dimes, and quarters needed to feed the machines. The wait could be an hour or longer. Fortunately, I soon learned a shortcut. A few isolated Xerox* machines wedged in various corners of the stacks were unknown to most people, and there was usually little or no wait.

I copied several tables and figures from the articles, summarized these in a few new tables, typed a series of short bullet points and conclusions, and delivered these to the art reproduction service in the basement of the hospital, where they were photographed as slides.

The weekly department-wide seminars at the Mass General were held in august surroundings, the famous Ether Dome, a sharply ascending amphitheater decorated with medical relics housed in old glass cases; there was even an Egyptian sarcophagus adjacent to the podium. The faculty sat up front, the most senior of them front row center, with trainees like me behind them and students in the back. Everyone wore white coats. I'd spoken here once before, on the anatomy of Parkinson's disease,

---

* The copying machines at Countway were foreign brands, but we still referred to them as Xerox machines.

but that had been a nightmare. There had been so much to learn, the content did not go down easily, and after being up all night, I was frazzled. My performance was mediocre at best. But this time I approached the task with confidence. There was great value in what I was proposing, and I believed that it would go well.

I approached the task with gusto, channeling my inner Dan Kemp back in room 10–250 at MIT. I began with a review of the history of therapies for MS. I ignored the nutty ones, and started with an injectable steroid treatment pioneered by Leo Alexander, a Boston neuropsychiatrist who had a private practice just down the block from our medical school.

Next, I discussed a low-dose chemotherapy medication that some physicians, including one at my hospital, had used,* noting that despite two decades of experience with this drug, I could find no evidence to indicate whether this approach had any value. Then, turning to the studies of Hommes and Gonsette, I highlighted their shortcomings. One really couldn't be sure if high-dose cyclophosphamide was helpful for MS. However—and this was the key—after reading these reports, it seemed exceedingly unlikely that the treatment would make MS worse.†

It was only near the end of my talk that I introduced the two patients who suffered from MS in addition to another condition that altered the activity of their immune systems, emphasizing that their stories supported the idea that turning off immunity could turn off MS. Two patients only, but powerful observations in sync with the claims of Hommes and Gonsette.

Before wrapping up, I stepped back to survey the broader

---

* Azathioprine, given daily by mouth.

† An important conclusion, because the maxim "first do no harm" is part of the Hippocratic oath taught to generations of medical students. However, if physicians only act to never cause harm, therapies that are beneficial on average will be withheld.

landscape of what was known about MS at the time. Theories were based on two competing concepts: one, that MS is caused by a viral infection; the second, that an autoimmune attack by an overactive immune system is responsible. If a virus causes MS, then immune suppression should make patients worse by weakening host defenses needed to fight the infection. However, if MS is an autoimmune disease, then suppressing immunity should be beneficial. My clinical experience indicated that the autoimmune cause is likely correct, and it was thus reasonable to undertake a well-designed study to try to confirm that infusions of high dose cyclophosphamide will benefit patients with MS.

* * *

As I made my way through the presentation, I occasionally looked up to scan the audience and was struck by their rapt attention and the more than occasional nod of agreement.

Best of all was the expression on Ray Adams's normally expressionless face: a simple raised eyebrow, which by now I knew signaled approval. After I finished, Adams spoke, as he normally did at the end of seminars at Mass General. A surprising comment.

"Charles Kubik and I reviewed the pathology in a large number of MS cases. In two, the lesions were just beginning to form, and in both the earliest change appeared to be ischemic damage; we found no lymphocytes in the brain in these early lesions," he explained. "Perhaps inflammation isn't the inciting event."

Translation: My trial might not be successful if the root of MS was inadequate blood flow, not autoimmunity or infection. If the lymphocytes that are present in the brain of every MS patient turn out to be merely the response to an injury, and not its cause, then cyclophosphamide would likely fail. Nonetheless, he still encouraged me to go forward with the trial, and made his comments in a contemplative, respectful, tone.

Almost as if we were peers.

CHAPTER 20

Origins of Autoimmunity

There was one other conclusion from my seminar, a private one not shared on any slide: I was flabbergasted that so little was actually known about the cause of MS, or for that matter any autoimmune disease. Explanations found in books were convoluted, some not much better than gobbledygook, and with more reading there was more uncertainty. Science should make the world easier to understand, but this was clearly not the case in MS. Testing cyclophosphamide was important, but it was also a superficial approach, a sledgehammer to address an intricate unknown disturbance in a complex biological system.

To make a meaningful contribution, I knew that I'd need to spend many years in basic science, in the lab. I was, in my mind, already becoming a physician-scientist, connecting medicine with basic research, but I also realized that the approaches to each were different. As a scientist I'd search for fundamental answers, but as a physician I had a responsibility to leave no stone unturned for my patients who can't wait for the complete answer to be uncovered—they need help immediately.

I branched out further, spending evenings and weekends in the lab when I wasn't on call with patients, consuming everything I could find about autoimmunity and MS. I wanted to catalogue what was known for sure, as well as what was uncertain or, worse yet, just opinion masquerading as fact. A starting point was the concept that our immune system evolved in environments not at all like those today, and that urbanization and new relationships with the microbial world around us could alter how our immune system worked. If true, then autoimmune disorders should be more common today than in earlier times and might even be a new health problem. How solid was, and is, the evidence?

To answer this question, I'd need to go back in time.

* * *

Before beginning this brief historical excursion, I should note that any attempt to reconstruct the early origins of autoimmune disease leads down a murky trail, fraught with uncertainty. This was true in the 1970s and remains the case today. Not much has changed, so for this trip I'll look at the evidence from today's perspective.

Medical paleontology, the study of ancient bones, offers a path. Bones resist decay. The rest of our bodies—brain, heart, lungs, liver, kidneys, guts—quickly decompose after death, and the trail of disease is lost forever. Unless, that is, the inflammation in the organs leaves its mark on the bones; or the death was by freezing and the body preserved in ice; or, more often, when the body was chemically treated, wrapped, and mummified. The nature of ceremonial burials varies, but the body is almost always laid in a position of repose, fingers and wrists in place. Many cultures, including our own, seem to have limited respect for the term "rest in peace."* So scientists can sometimes gain access to ancient bodies that are still intact. It might

* As a member of President Obama's Bioethics Commission, I was surprised to learn that many modern bioethicists believe that the right to privacy dies with the body. This is why famous historical figures can be exhumed, or their body parts probed with modern invasions, such as DNA testing of a sample of Lincoln's hair to search for evidence of Marfan syndrome, an inherited disease producing a tall and thin body frame and a propensity to aneurysms.

be possible to do an autopsy. Or if analysis of the bones will do the trick, get an X-ray, CT scan, or MRI.

There is an autoimmune disease for every organ in the body. Most organs have many, the brain dozens, and new ones are frequently uncovered. Some are quite rare, while others like MS are relatively common. And in addition to those that strike only a single organ in the body, others, like lupus and vasculitis, affect multiple different tissues. Altogether, more than one in ten people develop an autoimmune disease. And to estimate the frequency of autoimmune diseases in the past, the fossil record is most helpful for diseases that affect bones.

To look for evidence of inflammation in bones, rheumatoid arthritis should be as good as it gets. A common autoimmune disease that affects the joints at the edges of bones, rheumatoid arthritis is like MS in many ways, except of course that it inflames the joints rather than the brain. Because the damage is adjacent to bone, rheumatoid arthritis, of all the autoimmune diseases, is the one most likely to leave its mark. Bony erosions, small cavities where nodules of inflammation had silently drilled into the bone long ago, should be visible. And if the wrist and fingers are still with the skeleton, and not carried away for lunch by a possum or wild dog, they might display the characteristic twists and bends of rheumatoid arthritis.

Thousands of human remains have been scanned, probed, and chopped up over the years searching for signs of rheumatoid arthritis. Approximately 1 percent of the population suffers from the disease, so the fossil record should reveal many cases based on its frequency today. And while remains of the Egyptian royals Amenhotep III, Ramesses II and III, and Merneptah show clear X-ray evidence of spine disease that initially suggested rheumatoid arthritis, on closer analysis a different condition now seems much more likely.* So the story of bones tells us that rheumatoid arthritis was likely much less common in ancient times . . . if it was present at all.

Bones aren't the only historical record, of course. Humans have always communicated, always painted, and the written record could provide evidence of autoimmunity's path through the ages. There appear to be descriptions of arthritis by Hippocrates and other ancient observers, and rheumatoid hands seem to be depicted in young women in Renaissance paintings (such as Rubens's *The Three Graces*). But one cannot be sure; the descriptions are too imprecise, too primitive, and the images could equally represent artistic poses, old injuries, or other medical problems.

Autoimmune disease of the intestines—ulcerative colitis and its close neighbor Crohn's disease—are another common affliction. Ghastly symptoms: diarrhea with blood, abdominal cramps that make one bend over in pain and never want to straighten up. Diagnostically speaking, however, diarrhea is even less specific than joint symptoms. Intestinal maladies have plagued humankind forever, rumbling along in all seasons and then striking suddenly, killing millions in epidemics. Cholera, typhoid, simple food and water poisoning. Wars have more often been decided by intestinal disease than strategy, and even in the recent Gulf War, half of US servicemen suffered from diarrhea. So, amid this background of gastrointestinal disturbance as the norm throughout history, it's just not possible to conclude that an autoimmune cause was responsible for vague

* The bone disease diffuse idiopathic skeletal hyperostosis (DISH) is the current best guess to account for these findings; see S. N. Saleem and Z. Hawass, "Ankylosing Spondylitis or Diffuse Idiopathic Skeletal Hyperostosis in Royal Egyptian Mummies of 18th–20th Dynasties? CT and Archaeology Studies," *Arthritis & Rheumatology* 66 (2014): 3311–16.

descriptions of chronic diarrhea found in ancient or medieval texts.

And although details differ, the same uncertainties apply to the historical record of other autoimmune conditions, such as lupus, or those that affect the liver, kidneys, lungs, heart, muscles, or skin. Some things are just not knowable. Might as well ask your cat for the true story of what happened at Roswell.

* * *

And of all of these shadows of the past, the trail of MS might be the toughest to follow. No bones to scan here. No bodies of ancient climbers with MS, flash frozen by a sudden snowstorm on a Himalayan peak. Absent real data, we are left to rely on medical stories of illnesses as told at the time. And the conclusions deduced from these tales by contemporary writers are often subject to conjecture, wistful thinking, overinterpretation, and worse. Digging deep into junk rarely yields a diamond, but the topic is of such profound importance that even a smattering of data might illuminate the road ahead. Is MS a new disease, or has it been with us for centuries?

Lidwina was born in Holland in the late 14th century. At age 15, she fell while skating and fractured a rib. Afterward, it was said that she was bedridden with infections. She appears to have had weakness in her legs by age 19, but she may have recovered temporarily. Episodes of imbalance and further weakness pepper the narrative, and she ultimately went blind near the end of her life. She may also have had a progressive disease that left her able to move only her head and left arm at the time of death at age 53.

Several historians have concluded that Lidwina suffered from MS. Maybe, but she had other manifestations not typically seen. She completely avoided food except for small pieces of apple and dates, washed down with contaminated river water. She slept little or not at all. She bled from her mouth, nose, and ears, and sloughed off skin, bones, and intestinal matter that gave off a sweet smell and that were stored in a vase by her parents.

Lidwina also had mystical visions of heaven and hell, visited with Christ, and could cure those who came to her bedside. In 1890, she was anointed by Pope Leo XIII as the patron saint of ice skaters and the chronically ill. And each year in her hometown of Schiedam, a suburb of Rotterdam, on the second Sunday after Easter, the residents celebrate the life of this remarkable non-eater with an annual feast in her honor.

To a contemporary reader, the surviving accounts of Lidwina's life, her suffering, and her extraordinary gifts seem scriptural, a tragedy mixed with ten parts fantasy, imbued with the beliefs of the narrator. The medical history, moreover, is so primitively conveyed, so indistinct, so lacking in essential details as to be diagnostically useless.

* * *

The haze clears about 200 years ago, for MS and for many other medical conditions, as more systematic documentation of symptoms and the course of illnesses appear. The MS story begins with a royal family. But this time, it's not the pharaohs but the family of George III, King of England.

The illegitimate sixth son of the king's sixth son, the Earl of Essex, Augustus Frederick d'Este was by all accounts a spoiled and poorly behaved adolescent. As a young adult, he joined the military, adapting to the regimented structure, rising within the ranks, and ultimately participating in the Battle of New Orleans, an American victory that ended the War of 1812.

After peace was restored, Augustus returned to England. A lifelong bachelor, he would become deputy park ranger in London and a champion of the rights and welfare of aboriginal people, especially Native Americans. We know this in part because of the remarkable diary he maintained throughout his life. It is this diary that allows us to begin the trail of MS with Augustus.

In 1822, at age 28, he writes that he has developed an "indistinctness of vision" that prevents him from reading, yet his vision later recovers "without anything having been done to my eyes." Four years later, the symptom returns, and then remits again. Augustus next describes a constellation of neurologic problems, attacks followed by remissions and then, later on, permanent and progressively worsening symptoms: double vision, weakness in the legs, fatigue, burning pains, incontinence, and impotence. Fifteen years after onset he still experiences attacks and remissions, but is now also permanently weak and numb below the waist and has painful spasms in his legs. He eventually loses the use of his arms and dies in December 1848, 26 years after the onset of his disease.

There can be little question that Augustus suffered from MS. Initially his MS was the relapsing and remitting type, by far the most common way the disease begins, but after about 15 years, his illness gradually became progressive, in line with the typical course before effective therapy for MS was available.

Was Augustus the first person ever to be afflicted with MS, or was it Lidwina, or perhaps some ancient human or prehistoric hominid who lived centuries earlier? No diaries from Neanderthals exist, no frozen ancient bodies or preserved brain tissue revealing MS, and no hints found in the medical writings of the ancients. For now, the trail must begin with Augustus.

* * *

While we can't be sure that MS, or rheumatoid arthritis, or any other autoimmune condition, is a new disease, it's likely that MS, and others, have increased in frequency in recent years. Some of this rise is due to better recognition and diagnostic tests. Even when these advances are taken into account, however, there is little doubt that MS and other autoimmune diseases have become more prevalent.

Today, nearly 1 million Americans are known to have MS, a threefold increase in just one generation. Most of this change appears to be due to an increase in the number of women with the disease. A hundred years ago, both genders were equally affected, but today nearly three in four new cases occur in women.

Why has the risk in women exploded? One clue is that when MS begins in childhood, the number of cases in boys and girls are similar. Only at puberty does the excess risk to women first appear. This suggests that hormones play a critical role.* And puberty now occurs more than two years earlier on average than it did in the early 20th century, possibly because we eat more food than our ancestors and ingest additives such as steroids and antibiotics now common in our food supply.

These are not the only differences, of course. Women are more likely today to work outside the home, smoke, travel, attend college, have careers. But many of these features of modern life are also true for men. Family studies (in twins and non-twin siblings) have taught us that a critical exposure that sets the stage for MS occurs very early in life, maybe even before we are born. A second MS-predisposing event appears to take place later in childhood. Both events happen many years before MS begins. We still don't know exactly what the key ingredients are, but the

---

* Women are protected from MS attacks during pregnancy, especially during the second half of pregnancy, while the risk of attacks increases in the postpartum period. This is perhaps not surprising; it makes sense that the body's immune system would quiet down during pregnancy so that it does not attack the father's gene products, i.e., proteins, inherited by the fetus. In some animal models of MS, estrogens are protective against attacks, while progesterone may have the opposite effect. Prolactin, the milk-inducing hormone secreted during the postpartum period, can also worsen some models of MS. However, no single hormone can be clearly linked to the pregnancy and postpartum effects on MS activity.

trail is warm. MS is a medical mystery more exciting than any Sherlock Holmes caper.

So even if Augustus d'Este was not the first person to ever have MS, we know that in the early 19th century MS was likely much less common than it is today. Since our genes vary only slightly from one generation to the next, the only explanation for this modern epidemic is some change in the environment. And, as already seen, one thing that has changed is our longstanding relationship with germs.

* * *

I'll explain with an example close to home.

My Uncle Perry was a taxi driver in New Orleans. He was also a clean freak, one in a long line of excessive hand washers in our family, and someone who gradually placed so many restrictions on his customers that he put himself out of business.

No cigarettes. No cigars. No smokeless tobacco. No drinking. No eating. No chewing gum. Remove all of your trash—no waste to be left in the cab. Wipe your shoes before entering. Maximum three passengers. No children permitted in this taxi. Animals not allowed.

I'm also a germaphobe, a trait that runs through Mom's side of the family, but unlike Perry, I control it pretty well. Just a few simple daily rituals do the trick. Apart from a little bit of unnecessary handwashing, clothes changing, and office/closet cleanings, I've learned to limit the excesses so that my hands don't chafe. Loss of protective skin oils, a barrier against infection, can have dangerous consequences for physicians, increasing rather than decreasing the risk of infection.

I know that these are not rational behaviors, as the same bugs are everywhere. So they are best kept private, out of the public eye. But on occasion they can bubble up to the surface. This happened to me after my bachelor days were over and I became a parent for the first time.

When our firstborn was an infant, my parental instincts were on high alert. I was determined to protect my son against environmental germs—mostly imagined. My closest friends knew that even they could not touch the baby. I forced the poor babysitter to submit to frequent handwashing. Everything was sterilized, organic, pure. Teething biscuits were individually wrapped.

My growing list of rules for interacting with our little one soon became an object of good-natured ribbing by friends. I was turning our house into Perry's taxicab. In the laboratory where I worked, my name was now "Papa Steve." Even as our youngster advanced to a full diet, no processed foods were permitted; nothing artificial would touch his lips.

When our second child arrived, I let up a little bit. Looking back at old photographs, I see so many of my friends holding him, playing with him. And by the time that the third one came, I'd pretty much abandoned the hygiene fixation.

There was nothing specific—no flu, plague, or other infection—that I was trying to shield my kids against. I was just daddy hen with an overactive protective response.

I was ignoring my training as an immunologist. I knew that by inhibiting the natural development of my sons' immune systems, brilliantly guided by the pushes and pulls of environmental exposures over 7,000 earlier generations, I might upset the balance of its fine-tuning and produce more serious complications down the road. I was not considering the beneficial effects of early life exposure to infections.

The surface and openings and inner linings of our bodies are glazed with bugs—bacteria, funguses, parasites. We carry around more of their cells than our own. Our bodies are melting pots. We are colonized with intruders, and although we may think them uncouth and dirty, we need them. Some are recent settlers, but many are old friends who have been with us for millennia. They coevolved with us. And the hidden family secret is that we even mixed DNA. Our energy machinery, the mitochondria within our cells, came from them.

So we are all chimeras, mostly human but part bacteria. Whether they invaded us or we ingested them is a matter of perspective, but in any event, we've cohabitated for so long that separation is impossible. We can no longer survive without them. They carry out tasks that we're unable to do on our own. They help feed us; without their labors, we'd starve of essential nutrients that we cannot manufacture. And for every human gene in our body, we carry around more than 50 from bacteria whose products are constantly released in our bodies. About one in five proteins in our bloodstream is made by bacteria, not by us. They regulate our appetite, energy, mood, thinking. And there are even more viruses than bacteria living in us and on us.

Like us, the germs adapt and survive, and they do this by changing their DNA at a much faster rate than we can—500,000 times faster. Bacteria divide every 20 minutes, while we can only pass our genes to the next generation every 20 years or so. Seen from this perspective, humans are inflexible; we adapt slowly to new surroundings. We're also new to the scene. We go back less than 200,000 years, fewer than 8,000 generations, or about four one-thousandths of 1 percent of Earth's history. By contrast, bugs can go through 8,000 generations in less than three months.

Throughout most of human history, indeed until about 400 generations ago, we traveled in small groups, no larger than 10 to 20 people. Nuclear families linked by DNA, sharing similar bugs, not meeting many outsiders. Then, about 10,000 years ago, came agriculture and animal husbandry, and humans could settle down instead of wander as nomadic hunter-gatherers. We became homesteaders, farmers, and ranchers. A few could now produce and distribute food for many, sprouting colonies, villages, towns, cities, empires. For the first time, humans were now in contact with thousands of others, sharing our ideas, our art, our science, and our germs. And over the past 100 years, the changes have accelerated at a breakneck pace. We live in cities of millions, travel at 35,000 feet in flying metal cylinders where our germs mix with those of other passengers from across the globe, each one colonized by 500 trillion organisms. And through widespread use of vaccinations, antibiotics, pesticides, and food preservatives, we've discombobulated our long-standing symbiotic relationship with bugs. Turned it upside down.

Of all our body's tissues, our immune system is most dependent on the microscopic life forms that cohabitate with us. We've been engineered to operate in an equatorial forest of bugs. Without them, our immune defenses become soft, ineffective, unsuccessful.

* * *

One of my neighbors is a car nut, with money to burn—a dangerous combination. One fall afternoon, he took me on a drive in his new forest green Ferrari. It was baseball playoff season, and our steroid-powered San Francisco Giants were playing. I looked forward to listening to the play-by-play. After opening the door and contorting my body to get through the tiny opening and squirm into the ground-level passenger seat, I searched the dashboard for the radio. But, alas, it was nowhere to be seen.

"Where's the radio?"

"Don't have one. The engine is too loud to hear it anyway. The car is designed to immerse us in the sound of the engine, not music or talk."

The car could not climb any of the steep roads in our hilly

town because its aerodynamic bumpers, reaching nearly to the ground, would scrape against the concrete. The Ferrari was engineered to perform magnificently on a graded racetrack, where it could reach 200 miles per hour with no trace of vibration, but it failed miserably as a daily driver that could tune into the ballgame or navigate potholed streets.

Our immune system was sculpted over the eons, through trial and error and survival of the fittest, to work within a particular ecosystem. Change that ecosystem, and you can throw out evolution's improvements. Like the finely tuned Ferrari—perfection on a racetrack but useless on a hilly road—our lymphocytes work best when educated in the bug-filled world of our ancestors. With fewer or different bugs around, our immune system no longer works as intended.

* * *

During World War II, Allied troops stationed in Egypt experienced a terrible epidemic of paralytic polio. This was completely unexpected, as polio was unknown in this part of the world. Troops from the United States, Britain, and New Zealand, among other nations, had been deployed there to provide a wedge against incursions by the Axis powers, led by Hitler and Mussolini. Similar outbreaks occurred in other parts of the Middle East, North Africa, and the Philippines.

How could polio have broken out in areas that were untouched by the global epidemic? Where did the virus come from? How were the troops infected? And why were the locals spared? The answer soon came. The polio virus, far from being absent in Egypt, was ubiquitous. It was everywhere, in the pools and ponds, tap water rich with virus from human sewage, cocktails served at the military canteens, falafel sold on the street. It was transmitted with each handshake.

In 1943, as Egypt was invaded by Mussolini's forces, every

infant in Egypt had also been invaded . . . by the teeming, proliferating, replicating poliovirus. But they were protected by antibodies against polio, present in their bloodstream, transferred from their mothers in utero. Not lifelong protection, but something even better: a temporary shield from Mom until baby's immune system takes hold. A perfect solution, as if by divine plan.

Polio enters the baby's body through the mouth, travels down to the intestines, and multiplies there, causing pain, fever, and diarrhea. The baby is sick. For the virus, though, reaching the intestines is just the first step in its strategic plan—polio seeks total victory. The victim should be rendered helpless. And to do this, the virus must pass into the bloodstream, hitch a ride to the brain and nerves, penetrate and incapacitate them. Checkmate—permanent paralysis.

But the host, the baby, is prepared. Because baby's immunity is acquired "passively," from Mom, and not "actively" by its own immune system, antibodies are present in the bloodstream but nowhere else. The virus is permitted entry to the intestines, but when it passes through the walls of the intestines and into the bloodstream, it cannot survive—it's neutralized by Mom's antibodies, her unspoken gift to her baby for survival in a hostile world.

And it gets even better.

As the polio virus crosses over the intestinal wall, it also reaches the baby's immune system—the lamina propria, an enormous factory of immune cells conveniently located adjacent to the intestines where invaders are detected, sliced, diced, and presented on a platter. Within a few weeks, the infant's B cells are educated to make highly potent antibodies able to fight future infections should the virus ever reappear. Long-lasting, lifelong protection against polio.

So Mom's gift is a partial shield: it protects against paralysis but permits limited infection so that the baby can develop its own lifelong immunity. And this needs to happen within the first year of life, while Mom's passively transferred protection is still in the baby's bloodstream.

Our body's defense shield has been shaped over millions of years by the life forms present in the primeval muck, the drinking water and carrion ingested by our hunter-gatherer ancestors. Our immune system is essentially the same as theirs, but we now live in wildly different environments. It's not surprising that our ancient protective systems misfire. Maybe the only surprise is that this doesn't happen more often.

More than a century ago, H. G. Wells envisioned an alien invasion of Earth in his sci-fi classic *War of the Worlds* that was nearly successful but in the end was thwarted by microscopic domestic bugs, benign to Earthlings but lethal to the Martians. Like soldiers with polio or Indigenous people first encountering European measles, the Martians' immune system hadn't been trained through prior encounters, and they couldn't fight back against the germs.

* * *

We've seen that immune cells carrying receptors poised to attack the body's healthy tissues are not removed effectively unless bugs are present in sufficient abundance during early life. So with a cleaner environment, not only is the immune system less effective in fighting bugs but it is also more likely to turn against the home team.

One way that this can happen is when we disturb the ecosystem by removing bugs that have learned to dial down the host's defenses so that they are not destroyed. Without them, our immune system becomes overactive.

A study of people with highly active MS was underway in Buenos Aires when something unexpected happened. Some patients suddenly went into complete remission. They were not treated with any medication. But one thing had changed. Each had become infected with an intestinal tapeworm, and the body's immune response against the worm quieted the MS.*

The implications for people with MS were obvious, but almost nobody would choose to inoculate themselves with live worms that grow in the intestines to seven feet in length or longer, compete with the body for essential nutrients, infect loved ones, and invade other organs, including the brain.

Fortunately, other studies soon showed that dead worms had similar effects as living ones, and many patients began to treat themselves with freeze-dried tapeworm extracts. Over time, however, the benefits were disappointing, and the fad soon died out. But this discovery also paved the way for new research aimed at developing a novel class of anti-autoimmunity drugs based on potent molecules secreted by worms and other parasites that could turn off an immune attack against them.

* * *

Of all human maladies, autoimmune diseases provide the biggest challenge to our notions of biological superiority—the arrogant belief that we are here today, that our genetic lineage has survived across the eons, because we are the fittest beasts in the forest. What a disappointment! Our finely honed system of defense against bugs doesn't work as it should. It attacks us.

We're toast.

And the horror is even more profound when the attacker turns against the brain, against central command. At stake is our personhood, our very identity as sentient beings capable of creative thought, love, empathy, and generosity. One day we

---

* Immune cells can regulate, or turn down, immune responses in several ways. One powerful natural immune suppressant molecule is the protein interleukin-10 (IL-10), which is stimulated in the presence of the tapeworm.

are respected at work, beloved at home, a pillar of the community. The next, we're getting concerned glances because we've started behaving "out of character." Damage our heart, kidneys, or liver—we are still us. But take away our cognitive essence, and the substance of what makes us human has been lost. To lose all this, and to have been clobbered from within, is unthinkable. This is what happened to Andrea.

Fortunately, we've also been blessed with unique gifts—logic, creativity, and purpose—that give us a chance, maybe not to outwit these forces but to uncover basic principles of health and disease that can relieve suffering and make a huge impact in our lives; imperfect rear-guard actions to be sure, but potentially very consequential nonetheless. And for me, all that I'd learned about autoimmunity and MS could provide a runway to do exactly this—first, by testing the effects of cyclophosphamide in people with MS, and then, just maybe, down the road, by making a discovery that could pave the way for something far more effective.

CHAPTER 21

Love and Science

In the spring of 1979 I was a fourth-year resident, just a few months away from beginning my final year of clinical training, and with new responsibilities to supervise younger residents and teach students I felt ready for liftoff. My highest priority was to test whether cyclophosphamide had beneficial effects against MS. I asked for a review and approval from the Human Studies Committee of the Massachusetts General Hospital, which had recently been created to oversee human research and ensure that studies were carried out in a manner consistent with emerging ethical guidelines. After I presented the rationale and design for the study, they signed off, one of the first approvals that the new committee had granted.

A practical advantage of my study was that it wouldn't cost a cent in new funding. I simply wrote the treatment orders in the patients' charts and it was done, paid for by their insurance, something that would never be possible today.

* * *

I was slated that summer to begin a months-long rotation at the Fernald State School in Waltham, Massachusetts, a large residential campus and chronic care hospital for mentally and physically disabled people. But at this point I was consumed by my cyclophosphamide study, work with patients, evenings and weekends in the lab, and thought that my experiences as a medical student—the year studying autism and working at Belchertown—had already given me sufficient grounding so that a Fernald rotation was unnecessary. One evening, I met one of my colleagues, Ed Zalneraitis, in the hospital lobby.

"Ed, I'm going to tell Dr. Adams tomorrow that I need to be excused from Fernald," I said. "I have too much going on here."

"OK," he replied, "but if I were you, I'd give it a try, at least for a day or two. There's a pediatric resident who's just starting her rotation there. She's from California. She's beautiful, tall, and really nice. I've been telling her all about you. You'll really like her, but the two of you are very different. She may be too much of a hippie for you."

I took the bait.

Our eyes met as I walked out of the elevator at Fernald's conference room, arriving at the last minute for a seminar that I was participating in. Elizabeth recalls first noticing my starched white shirt and perfectly knotted tie and thinking, *He looks so clean.* I remember saying to myself, *My goodness, Ed was right*, and also that her hair looked slightly wet, due, I'd later learn, to an early morning swim in the icy waters of Revere Beach.

We had coffee together after the seminar, enough time for me to ask her out. She said yes.

Fantastic.

On that first date, we found out that we both loved the same Cat Stevens and Ella Fitzgerald albums. We also soon realized that these shared affinities were the exceptions. Ed Zalneraitis was right; we had almost nothing in common. We were poles apart politically. I'm a neat freak, while her blue Volkswagen Beetle hadn't been washed in years, and the back seat was stacked with old papers, food wrappers, and possibly worse. I'm a spendthrift, while she has little interest in material things. I'm a loner; she's an extrovert.

Fortunately, opposites attract.

We were soon an item. I also enjoyed Fernald. I still cared deeply about disabled people—I enjoyed interacting with them and helping as best I could. Soon I even had a job moonlighting as an on-call physician there, mostly night and weekend work. Elizabeth would often join me, bringing picnic dinners from DeLuca's Market on Charles Street that we'd eat together, lakeside, at nearby Wellesley College. During the week, we'd share meals at Fernald's cafeteria, surrounded by a bevy of institutionalized residents who'd smile and laugh and occasionally grunt, or say a few words to us.

Several weeks later, Elizabeth was walking down one of the long hallways of Massachusetts General Hospital when she was stopped by Dr. Fisher.

"Do I hear wedding bells?" he asked with a wry smile.

They'd never met, and only a few of our best friends even knew we were dating.

* * *

My cyclophosphamide study was now launched, and I planned to recruit 40 patients, half of whom would receive cyclophosphamide intravenously for a two-week period (the exact duration of treatment would depend on each individual's response to the drug). It was a big undertaking; each patient would need to be hospitalized for several weeks at least, and the intensive treatments reduced the body's protective immunity for a short period of time, creating a risk for serious infection. So each patient needed to be carefully monitored, 24–7. Several fellow residents and even faculty agreed to assist with patient care, and without this team I wouldn't have been successful. But this was my baby, and I'd take personal responsibility for every detail. Before enrolling a patient, I'd spend hours discussing every aspect of the study, reviewing all possible risks, emphasizing the uncertainty of any benefit, and also reassuring them that I'd remain available to help them even if they decided not to participate. Sometimes I'd go through the discussion multiple times, with repeat sessions for family members. Each patient would be a partner in the study, and it was essential that they understood exactly what they were getting into.

The plan was to enroll patients over a two-year period, and then it would take an additional two years of observation to see if cyclophosphamide changed the course of MS—an agonizingly long wait. And as I waded into my first clinical study, something else was already becoming clear: simply testing drugs that others had reported as effective was inadequate for the sort of career I was now envisioning.

To really understand MS, I had to know more about the basic biology of the immune system, the cells that caused my asthma and eczema and now also inflamed the brain of my patients. As a physician, I could try to treat patients with toxic therapies. I'd already started down that path. But to do something more substantial, I'd need to master the science of autoimmunity.

* * *

The story of autoimmunity arose in the shadow of vaccination as its evil twin. It began with the long-ago observer, lost to history, who first noticed that survivors of epidemics tended to be resistant to future ones. This simple, profound discovery is one of the most meaningful in the history of medicine.*

During the Middle Ages, it was common practice to intentionally expose healthy people to individuals with mild cases of smallpox—by spending time in close proximity, sharing contaminated blankets, or scratching pus through the skin—

---

* Rivals for this title are the germ theory of disease (1861), anesthesia (1846), and antibiotics (1928).

transferring a similarly mild illness to recipients in order to protect them from future outbreaks. Throughout the 18th century, vaccination was practiced throughout much of Europe and in colonial America. It was observed that milkmaids exposed to cowpox—a skin rash on the udders of dairy cows—were also resistant to smallpox, although it took until the end of the century for Edward Jenner to show that intentional vaccination with cowpox was a safe method to protect against smallpox. Exactly how vaccination worked was unknown, although there was speculation that "invisible animals" were responsible for epidemics long before Antonie van Leeuwenhoek peered into a microscope to see bacteria for the first time.

But vaccination could also produce terrible complications, and not only by causing the infection it was intended to prevent. Some recipients of Louis Pasteur's vaccine against rabies virus* developed devastating neurologic illnesses—confusion, paralysis, even death. There was massive brain swelling and the spinal cord was destroyed, turned to mush. It was first thought that rabies must be the culprit, but when the brain tissue was examined under the microscope, the pattern of damage was unlike any known rabies infection. Lymphocytes poured out of the bloodstream and into the brain, but they were not attacking nerve cells, as expected with rabies. Rather, they were encircling the protective insulating substance that surrounds nerve cells, the myelin membranes, and destroying them, a type of damage known as "demyelination." This never happens with rabies . . . but it does with MS!

It soon became clear that vaccination could cause demyelination, even when using dead rabies virus that had been grown in brain tissue or, shockingly, by injecting normal, healthy

---

* Live rabies virus was attenuated, or weakened, by passage of human extracts to rabbits, followed by inoculation of rabbit spinal cord tissue into humans.

brain tissue containing no virus at all. At first, it was thought that some undetected virus or toxin must have been hiding in the healthy brain tissue. After all, the founders of immunology taught us that our body's defense system could never attack itself.* So the brain inflammation was called "allergic," implying that the body was responding to some invader, perhaps an invisible bug hiding in the brain. Myelin must have been a bystander to the attack, injured by mistake. Autoimmunity†—an attack on the body's own myelin—was impossible.

Later, more cases of demyelination would occur in people vaccinated with inactivated measles virus and other viruses grown in brain tissue. Rare events all, and on balance each of these vaccines would produce far more good than harm.‡ Over time, it became clear that the brain tissue itself was responsible for firing up the immune attack. And soon it was recognized that the brain was not an exception; almost any tissue, ground up and injected under the right conditions, could also provoke a specific inflammatory reaction in the body. This led to the development of a large catalogue of autoimmune disorders in lab animals, most often mice: tissue from pancreas to produce diabetes, or collagen from joints for rheumatoid arthritis, or myelin from the brain for MS.

---

* At the dawn of the 20th century, the great immunologist Paul Ehrlich argued that immune reactions against one's own tissues were impossible, a concept that stood for nearly half a century despite the clear demonstration by Julius Donath and Karl Landsteiner in 1904 that autoimmune reactions against red blood cells could follow infection with syphilis.

† Called "horror autotoxicus" by Ehrlich.

‡ An exception is the polio epidemic caused by the Cutter vaccine in 1955. Modern vaccines have an outstanding track record for value and safety, but this is little consolation to the unfortunate few still injured by rare complications. And fear of lawsuits might cripple vaccine development. To protect the pipeline of new vaccines critical to advancing public health, the US government passed the National Childhood Vaccine Injury Act (1986), providing a ceiling on compensation for individuals injured through vaccine-related events. Unfortunately, vaccination phobias remain prevalent in some segments of society, fueled by unsubstantiated fears, religious beliefs, and conspiracy theories. And vaccines don't cause autism.

The immunized mice soon became standard disease "models" for deciphering the analogous human conditions; the immune cells responsible for disease could easily be determined, and effects of treatments efficiently tested, in genetically identical rodents housed in small cages on the benchtops of laboratories worldwide.

As recently as the 1970s, the mouse researchers, who were the overwhelming majority in the field, considered human immunology second-class science. People were too complex; there were so many variables to control, and results were often difficult to replicate. Our immune systems change dramatically, even over the course of a normal day, with more or less sleep, with diet, medication, and stress. Mice are easier than people. The critters are genetically identical; you can manipulate them in tightly controlled environments without asking their permission; and they don't miss clinic visits because of snowstorms or childcare issues. Mouse work is quicker, and results are more likely to stand the test of time.

Thus, our knowledge of autoimmune disease grew directly out of complications grounded in the vaccine experience and studies of disease mechanisms inferred from inbred mice.

As we'll soon see, this approach gave rise to enormous progress . . . along with misconceptions and oversimplifications.

Experimental allergic (or autoimmune) encephalomyelitis (EAE), first described by Thomas Rivers in 1932, has for nearly a century been the principal method used to study brain inflammation in the lab. Early experiments relied on the injection of either ground-up whole brain or isolated myelin tissue to produce EAE.

With refinements in chemistry, it was found that use of purified proteins, or even fragments of a single protein, could also do the trick—advantages included more focused immune reactions and greater reproducibility. One special myelin protein, an abundant one known as myelin basic protein (MBP), could reliably induce EAE in many animal species, and by the 1970s, MBP-induced EAE had become the gold standard for studying brain inflammation, and MS. In lab parlance, EAE is often referred to as a "model" for MS, meaning that it mimics some features of the human disease.

When mice are injected just underneath the skin with MBP that's been whipped up in a blender,* the immune system fires up. It begins with the local militia, gluttonous antigen-presenting cells, which live in the neighborhood and are on constant patrol for foreigners, outsiders, things that don't belong, things that are "not me." Once they detect something strange, they gobble it up and digest it, like goats. Then they call for the army—the lymphocytes—by releasing chemicals that drive lymphocytes wild, attracting them to the disturbance, the injection site, like bees to honey. The antigen-presenting cells display on their surface fragments of the foreign substances they've ingested, which are attached to proteins that only lymphocytes can see.† And rare lymphocytes, maybe one in a million, that recognize a fragment exactly, attach tightly, like a snap closure. They turn on, tune in, and proliferate, and are deployed throughout the body to search for other, identical, invaders. And if ground-up MBP was injected in the first place, the search finds its target in the nervous system. Lymphocytes flood in, myelin is attacked, and the mouse develops paralysis, visual loss, and other signs of brain disease.

A generation of young immunologists built their careers on EAE. It was a machine for generating data suitable for publication, and publications are the currency of science. Scien-

---

* Mixed with oil and dead fragments of tuberculosis to better stimulate the immune response.

† As we'll see in a later chapter, these are the major histocompatibility complex (MHC) proteins, which are a major factor in autoimmunity.

tists working in the pharmaceutical industry could screen large portfolios of drugs, every chemical on the shelves, to look for those that control EAE and propose them as treatments for MS.

Unfortunately, researchers sometimes seemed to forget that mouse EAE was not human MS, and this mindset would not change even after, time and again, treatments that cured the mice were found to be useless in people.

* * *

Across town from Mass General, at the Harvard Medical School quadrangle, was a young neurologist named Howard Weiner, only five years older than me, who was in the process of completing his training and ready to set up an immunology laboratory to study MS.

We hit it off. Howard had begun to treat MS patients with a blood-cleaning procedure, called plasma exchange, to remove toxic proteins in the bloodstream. We decided to merge our two studies together—mine with cyclophosphamide and his with plasma exchange. We'd still need 20 patients in each group, but it would be far more efficient to test both treatments together because we could share the same untreated control group. And furthermore, we'd be able to compare the two treatments against each other. I also decided to work in his new laboratory. Thus began a collaboration, and a friendship, that has lasted more than 40 years.

Science is a highly competitive, tension-packed activity. Every scientist frets over the possibility of being scooped, or worse yet publishing something later found to be wrong, and one needs friends to make it through the bumps in the road. Howard and I became brothers in science after that first meeting. We've worked together in studies of immunology, genetics, and therapeutics and served as mutual support systems as well as sounding boards for each other's ideas.

CHAPTER 22

A Key Insight

One of the pleasures of residency at Mass General was the opportunity to attend intimate research seminars with our chief, often given by people hoping to join our department. On a cool fall day in 1979, the presenter was a young researcher from MIT.

His subject was an analysis of the tissue changes he'd found in mouse EAE. As he described the paralysis he'd seen following injection of MBP (the myelin protein thought to possibly trigger autoimmunity in MS), it became clear that he'd missed a key problem with his results.

The room had not missed the problem, however, and started to turn against him. Ray Adams was impatient with data that he didn't respect, and knowing our boss well, we could all see his shifting posture and the facial tics that generally preceded the skewering that was about to take place.

"The paralysis you observed is due to peripheral nerve disease," Adams corrected the young researcher. "But MS doesn't cause peripheral nerve disease."

It was over. The seminar was a bust, and the speaker was put on notice to look for employment elsewhere.

Adams's comment was a critical insight. MS is caused by damage to myelin. As mentioned, that's the fatty substance that wraps around nerve cells, ensheathing them and preventing short-circuiting of transmissions in the brain. There are two types of myelin: one found in the brain and spinal cord of the central nervous system and the other in peripheral nerves that innervate arms and legs and other organs of the body.

In MS, only brain and spinal cord myelin is damaged. Peripheral nerves are spared. Any true model for MS should reflect this fact, but the study presented in this long-ago seminar failed the test because the immune system had attacked peripheral nerves.* I was amazed that this EAE model, the gold standard used to study MS in labs everywhere, could be so fundamentally defective.

That was not all; there was another huge problem with the EAE model. There was lots of inflammation throughout the brain, but damage to myelin was quite sparse. In fact, it was pretty subtle. On closer inspection, it really didn't look much like MS at all. In MS, the loss of myelin is by far the most conspicuous feature; it is dramatic, consisting of many oval or circular patches that pockmark the brain like Swiss cheese. MS myelin looks like it was hit by a nuclear bomb.

After the conference, I spoke with my boss.

"Dr. Adams," I asked, "do you think it's possible to develop a better model for MS?"

"Yes," he replied, "you should begin by looking at the old literature on EAE in monkeys. I've reviewed a number of these cases myself and was impressed by their close resemblance to acute MS lesions. They were much more convincing than anything I've seen in a mouse or other rodent."

Adams was recommending that I study monkeys instead of mice, but the thought of working with monkeys was beyond unattractive to me. I had ethical concerns about experimenting

---

* MBP is located in both types of myelin, central and peripheral. For this reason, inflammation triggered against MBP in the EAE model damaged both the central and peripheral nervous systems.

with animals that are phylogenetically close to humans. And the cost of working with nonhuman primates was also outside the budget of most young scientists. But beyond these ethical and practical considerations, there was an additional scientific problem. Primates were known to develop only short-lived, acute disease and not the chronic, long-lasting inflammation that was characteristic of human MS.

Despite my reservations and the many challenges that I'd face, I thought it might be possible to develop a valid MS model someday. I stored these thoughts away, not to retrieve them until nearly a decade later.

My off-hours work with Howard Weiner had gone exceedingly well. In addition to the cyclophosphamide study that we were now doing together, his lab provided me free rein to develop two projects, one using immune cells from MS patients, and the other using immune cells from mice with EAE. Two sides of the coin: I'd study people with MS—the real deal—and also the mouse facsimile. This was my first dive into lab research. I wanted to measure the sensitivity of lymphocytes to MBP in patients with MS and compare their responses with those of immunized EAE mice. This was one test of the validity of the mouse model. First, I'd have to prepare MBP. I jotted down the recipe, it really was cookbook style, jogged to the local butcher shop for a cow brain, returned to the lab where I ground it up in a Waring blender, followed the steps to extract the MBP, and lyophilized the final product to a white powder.

In the morning, bright and early, I'd draw blood from my patients and then from myself, a healthy control. Drawing one's own blood is the best way to learn the art of painless phlebotomy. Next, using another recipe, I prepared the lymphocytes, B cells, and T cells, pipetted them into test tubes, added a tiny amount of MBP, and then placed them in 37°F incubators for three days. I then quantitated how many times they divided, a measure of stimulation.

Lymphocytes from the mice with EAE divided like wildfire when cultured with MBP, up to 50 times more than normal, not surprising because I'd previously stimulated their immune systems with injections of MBP under the skin. The patients with MS had only a tiny bit of stimulation, much less than the mice, though, about one and a half times above the normal range. But my lymphocytes were the clear winner—when they were exposed to MBP they went into hyperdrive, dividing nearly a hundredfold!

How was this possible? I didn't have EAE, or MS for that matter. By preparing the MBP from the cow's brain, I must have inhaled tiny flecks of brain material in the dusty samples that I weighed, dried, dissolved, and injected into mice. An occupational exposure, one that I'd later confirm in other lab workers, but fortunately entirely benign. Not all lymphocytes that react against brain tissue are bad actors; some are neutral, others even confer protection.

Sorting out the cause of MS would be no simple task.

* * *

In 1980, at the age of 30 years, I finally completed my residency and had become a full-fledged internist and neurologist. My next move was a no-brainer. I'd move across town, to the main campus of Harvard Medical School, and begin a three-year postdoctoral research fellowship under Howard Weiner's direction. Soon after my arrival, Dr. Richard Tyler, the head of neurology at Harvard's Brigham and Women's Hospital,* asked me to establish a dedicated clinic for patients with MS, an opportunity that I accepted

---

* Strictly speaking, it was still called the Peter Bent Brigham Hospital, but the name would change later that year.

with gratitude and gusto. It was a great opportunity to bring together clinical medicine with biomedical investigations to try to learn more about MS.

There were many advantages to the move. I'd be at the center of a large community of immunologists, and Elizabeth had also secured a postdoctoral position at Harvard's cancer center just across the street from my lab. Moreover, I'd be reunited with medical school classmates who were also training there, and with one in particular, Norman Letvin.

Norman was a genius, but he was too close a friend for me to notice. His childhood was patrician, filled with classics and music academies. He hung out with Yo-Yo Ma, for goodness' sake. We were unalike in so many ways, but shared a sense of the ridiculous, fierce loyalty to our friends, and passion for what we were doing. We were in it for the right reasons. We wanted to cure disease and were enthralled by the study of how immune defenses ward off infections and cancer, but can also turn against the body itself to cause autoimmune disease.

Science was our bond, as we were poles apart in affinities and talents. Norman was a classically trained clarinetist, a prodigy, possessed of both skill and will. As a student in Boston, when short on cash, he'd hop the train to Manhattan for weekend gigs in the orchestra pit of Broadway musicals. "The music is brain-dead," he quipped. "I just show up and follow the score. No need to see it in advance."

Norman was a postdoc like me, but he worked at the largest immunology laboratory in the medical school, led by the head of the department. It was a pressure cooker, unlike the relatively relaxed environment of Howard's lab where I ran my own show. But the intellectual environment there was rocket propelled, and I enjoyed visiting, mostly to savor the scene in small doses, see Norm, and touch base with a few other classmates.

We'd have far-ranging discussions together, about MS, autoimmunity, and the value of EAE. "MS is caused by a virus," he'd say. "Autoimmune diseases are caused by infections. The EAE papers are all written by idiots. We can blow them out of the water."

"Norm, nobody has ever seen a virus in an MS brain. A virus could be the initial trigger, but I don't believe that it's still in the body when people are having MS attacks."

Although we disagreed, his passion and self-confidence were simply amazing to me.

And we set out to make an impact in the field. We'd work together in my lab, where there was plenty of space and nobody looking over our shoulder. We could order everything we needed without asking permission. My connection with Norm also meant that I'd be able to perform the most sophisticated experiments possible, as he worked at the best mouse immunology lab in the world. This level of work would not have been possible in my mentor's lab. We just didn't have the reagents—the raw materials—for the state-of-the-art immunology that was needed. But with Norman's help, we could bring everything we needed to my small lab and get to work.

Ray Adams had convinced me that mouse EAE was flawed as a model of human MS, but at the time there were no practical alternatives for serious lab investigations. And the model could still be quite useful. With new tools at our disposal, it should be possible to decipher with greater precision exactly which immune cells were responsible for brain inflammation in the EAE mice. T cells—the most abundant type of lymphocyte and the one capable of killing other cells—had to be the central actors, everyone knew that,* but maybe other cells also played a role.

---

* Our B cell studies that would overturn this notion would occur more than a decade later.

Here's why we thought that T cells caused EAE. In 1961, an ingenious scientist named Phil Paterson showed that he could remove T lymphocytes from a mouse with EAE and inject them into a genetically identical healthy mouse. Because the mice were identical, the transplanted T cells from the ill donor would be fully functional in the healthy recipient. Paterson found that the transferred T cells produced EAE in the recipient. Only T cells could do this.

Norman and I plotted out an experiment to look at the role of T cells in a different way. We'd destroy the entire immune system of the mouse by surgically removing the thymus gland and subjecting the animal to high doses of radiation, leaving it without immunity. All the cells needed for defense, the T cells and B cells, along with other white blood cells known as monocytes and leukocytes, were completely undetectable. We then immunized the mice with brain tissue, which would cause EAE in normal mice. Not surprisingly, these animals with no immune system were now resistant to EAE; they developed no inflammation or paralysis. Next, we transferred back the entire immune system except for T cells, and the mice still remained resistant. Finally, we transferred back T cells, and when the mice were immunized with brain tissue, they developed rip-roaring disease. This confirmed that T cells, presumably acting alone, could cause EAE. Case closed. Or so I thought.

* * *

The mega lab in which Norman toiled was tightly organized into units, each run by a favored lieutenant. The units were assigned similar projects, and the lieutenant that found the answer first would publish the career-making paper, win the accolades, and ascend to the next rung of Harvard's ladder. Not surprisingly, any progress that one group made was seldom shared with the others. Unit leaders had weekly one-on-one meetings with the boss, invariably followed by cracks of the whip and warnings to underlings to move faster.

The rules fostered productivity, but at a price. The environment was toxic. Siloed lab teams were unwilling to share technical advice, and rumors of sabotage swirled around failed experiments. It was dog-eat-dog, survival of the fittest.

One particularly unpopular junior faculty member became ill, first with fatigue, then numbness—beginning in the toes, then rising to the legs, arms, torso, and face—followed by weakness. He was hospitalized, and laboratory tests indicated only a mild liver disturbance. Neurologic testing showed that his reflexes were absent, and electrical studies pointed to damage in the peripheral nerves. A clear case of Guillain-Barré syndrome, taught to every medical student: an autoimmune disease caused by an attack on the myelin of peripheral nerves as they exit the brain and spine.* Guillain-Barré is often triggered by some sort of infection, and his fatigue and liver abnormalities were attributed to a virus.

Muscles of the chest wall are weakened with Guillain-Barré, and breathing is frequently compromised, so patients require urgent monitoring in intensive care units until the storm passes. With care, our colleague gradually stabilized, but he did not recover as quickly as expected. Several months later, his recovery was still only marginal, but he was able to accommodate the weakness in his feet and hands, adapt to the numbness, and return to work. However, a few weeks later, he suffered a relapse more severe than the first episode.

Analysis of his tissues revealed that he'd been poisoned with acrylamide, a laboratory chemical that was also traced to the coffee machine in his office. An investigation of the poisoning

* Guillain-Barré syndrome is a cousin to MS. Both are autoimmune diseases, but in MS, the myelin within the brain and spinal cord is inflamed, while in Guillain-Barré only the myelin outside of these areas is involved.

focused on a disgruntled student in the lab as the primary person of interest, but no proof could be found, and after some time, the case was dropped.

For the next few years, the running joke in the lab was to offer visitors a cup of coffee.

* * *

Norman appeared to be thriving despite the pressure, and we were making great progress in our work together across the two labs, trying to unravel how the immune system produced disease in our mouse model of MS. That is, until one day, when Seiji Ozawa, conductor of the Boston Symphony Orchestra and a living legend, came to the lab with a job offer. Norman had a rare gift, and with this gift came an obligation to pursue music. He should abandon science and join the symphony.

We had lunch the next day. Norman was rattled, caught between two incompatible worlds. He'd spoken with the big lab chief—a rare visit to Mount Olympus. "I told him about the symphony offer," he said. "You won't believe this. He told me he wanted me to stay in his lab. He even complimented me. He said that my work was great. He never compliments anybody. And he offered me a job! If I agree to stay until July, then he'd give me a faculty position with a lab, a salary, and startup research funds."

Now the playing field was level. Two secure offers, each an outstanding opportunity to breathe the most rarefied air at the summit of human creative work. Which would it be—music or science?

By Monday morning, he'd made his decision: "It was easy. Science is the higher calling."

Six months later, Norman returned to Olympus to settle on the details of his new job, but was now told that no position was in the offing.

"Your work, taken together, isn't worth five cents," the lab chief told him.

Nothing else had changed. The lab had needed Norman to complete his project, and the chief would say whatever was required to keep the ship on course.

Within a few weeks of receiving the bad news, Norman regrouped and was offered a position to lead an immunology effort at the Harvard-affiliated primate center located outside of Worcester, Massachusetts. He would have that coveted Harvard faculty title, but to us, Worcester may as well have been Siberia. To Norman, however, it was a new challenge.

"The animals are dying there of an unknown illness causing wasting, infections, and tumors," he explained to me. "Their scientists are idiots, and they don't have a clue. I think that I can solve this. It has to be a virus—don't you think?"

Great people find opportunity that others fail to see. Norman would go on to discover the monkey AIDS virus, the ancestor of human HIV, make giant contributions in understanding how the virus disables the body's immune system, and lead the world's effort in developing an AIDS vaccine. Eagles will soar.

And one more thing. If I had Norman's music gene and could play rock 'n' roll like Eric Clapton . . . and if Ed Sullivan had visited me in the lab . . . I'm not sure I'd have made the same choice.

CHAPTER 23

Loss and Launch

It came out of the blue. I knew that my dad was having "stomach troubles." A couple of years earlier, he had a colonoscopy that showed "a spasm." He said it was a horrible experience and he would never go through it again. He'd jump out of planes with bullets flying, but a colonoscopy was more than he could handle. He was 55 years old, athletic and fit, still a tough guy. The only health problem he'd ever had, except for the war injuries, was the time a few years back when he'd shattered his leg in a bicycle crash.

The call was from Mom: "Dad is in the hospital. The doctors think he has cancer. Don't come, you have so much on your mind."

I was there the next morning. Dad had just come out of emergency surgery to relieve a bowel obstruction. They'd found colon cancer, and he'd need a second operation to remove the tumor.

Lives can change in a flash.

I called William Silen, my former professor and the best GI surgeon anywhere. His textbook on abdominal disease was a classic, used by medical students around the world.

"Dr. Silen, my dad just had decompression of a bowel obstruction. They're pretty sure that he has colon cancer. Would you be able to take care of him?"

Within a few days, my folks were in Boston, Dad at the hospital while Mom stayed with Elizabeth and me—we'd moved into a small Beacon Hill apartment. The surgery to remove the main tumor was a success, but Silen found widespread metastases. He didn't share this news with any of us. He told Dad that he thought he got all of it, but just in case, he'd need chemotherapy. Just to be sure.

Dad healed. But he said he no longer felt strong. He was always tired; his head wasn't clear. Maybe lingering effects of the surgery and chemo, we thought. Dad mostly seemed fine. He and Mom crammed a lifetime of wanderlust into the next year. They traveled, hiked, camped, and biked, gazed at stars and lakes and mountains, did all of the things that they loved. But then the dwindles took over. Food was no longer enjoyable. Dad began to lose weight and was increasingly confined to the neighborhood, then our house, then his bed. And the belly pain was the worst part. Ten out of ten pain that increased to eleven whenever he tried to eat anything or drink even a few sips of liquid. Pain that made sleep impossible, life not worth living.

Dad saw an oncologist in New York who did a few tests. He rapidly diagnosed advanced terminal cancer and recommended higher doses of chemotherapy, mostly to try to reduce the pain.

I asked Dr. Silen what we should do. Did he know that my dad had metastases?

"Well, I thought that his liver felt hard," he said. "Your parents had a good year together, and they had hope that maybe everything would be OK."

Silen knew that there was nothing to be gained by sharing this news. Looking back, I think that he was right in my dad's case, although withholding essential health information today would be considered improper.

Every weekend when not on call, Elizabeth and I would drive the 220 miles from Boston to Queens to see Dad and help

Mom as best we could. Elizabeth would wake up early to make Dad an apple pie, his favorite, and one of the few foods that still appealed to him.

Dad was no match for this cruel disease. It rapidly marched through him, through the chemo. Within two years, he'd lost nearly half his weight. Everyone knew that the end was near. It was a new year, 1983, and our final visit. We went to Dad's sick room to share special news.

"Dad, Elizabeth and I wanted to tell you that we're going to get married."

"This is such wonderful news," he said. "I'm so happy. I've been hoping for this for a long time. And I have something to ask of you."

"Of course, Dad, anything."

"Please take care of your mother."

"I will, Dad. I promise."

Tears and hugs, and an apple pie party in Dad's room.

He died a few weeks later, in the middle of winter. The worst part was that I had to tell Grandpa Lou that his son had died. We hadn't told him that Dad was sick. My father asked that we keep his illness private; the news would sadden his father too much, Dad said, and could worsen his heart condition. He'd never recover from the news of Dad's death. For the second time I witnessed a parent bury a child in our family.

* * *

The first patient I treated with cyclophosphamide was Pete Smith, a tough-talking Vietnam vet from Revere, Massachusetts. He was only 25 but seemed older. It wasn't just the desperado mustache and thick black hair or the five o'clock shadow, it was that Pete had lived so much in a short time. The war had been tough, so many around him had died, and then at age 19 the MS arrived. With a bang. Attack after attack. Each day he'd struggle to walk, even though he'd only leave the wheelchair for a few halting steps, leaning dangerously forward on the forearm crutches, legs encased in the painful metal exoskeletons.

A sweet guy. Said he'd do anything to help others with MS so that they wouldn't have to share his fate.

As soon as the cyclophosphamide study began, I asked Pete if he'd like to enroll. "Of course, Doc. I'll do anything. I can't keep living like this."

When people are desperate, they might grasp at any thread of hope. Balancing hope with reality is always a challenge in medicine, but its importance is magnified in medical research. And when the scientist is also the treating physician, there is a particularly knotty conflict of interest. If we're being honest, the physician has a mixture of motives—good ones involving scientific discovery, solving medical problems, and allowing patients to lead much better lives. But there are also personal ones involving ambition and the rewards that come with success. And so it requires a high degree of transparency and self-reflection to find the best path forward.

I was confident that Pete was a good candidate for the study, but wanted to make sure that he fully understood the substantial risks of cyclophosphamide, including the possibility of life-threatening infection or even bladder cancer down the road. Equally important, he needed to know that the benefits, if any, would most likely be modest; if successful, his condition might stop worsening, but he would still be in a wheelchair. I also had lengthy meetings with his wife and parents, emphasizing that this was an aggressive approach to MS, and not something that Pete should take lightly.

When we selected his treatment from a bowl filled with folded papers, each containing the name of one of the three possible options, the paper read "cyclophosphamide."

And in rapid order, other patients signed on. The entire study consisted of 58 patients treated at the two Boston hospitals, Mass

General and the Brigham. I knew each patient, knew their loved ones, their stories. I shook their hands, thanked them for participating, for having confidence in us. Everything was recorded in a single spiral notebook. This was before computers, big data, MRIs, or treatments for MS.

It would take four years before we'd finally have full results of the trial to see if a chemotherapy drug that suppressed the immune system could help people with MS. I'd already seen evidence that it seemed to work in some patients. The final results showed that cyclophosphamide stopped MS from getting worse, convincingly. For almost a year, even longer in some patients. But unfortunately the benefit was only temporary. After 9 to 12 months, in some the MS kicked in again. We had hoped that it might be gone, but it was still there, lurking in the shadows and waiting to explode again. It was awful when we began to see, in patient after patient, that the respite was only temporary.

Flowers for Algernon by Daniel Keyes is the story of a drug that seemed to reverse mental retardation. In the book Charley is cured, and he heads for a new life filled with promise and happiness. But then the drug's effects wear off. The book suggests that Charley would have been better off not having experienced the transient benefit and false hope that all would be well.

My patients didn't feel this way, though. They saw the time in remission as a gift. And further, we found that they could take the drug again to lengthen the remissions, though after a few doses the cumulative risks—sterility and possibly cancer—become too great to continue.

Pete, sadly, was not one of the successes. His MS brushed off the cyclophosphamide as if it were a gnat. He later told me, "Doc, even though it didn't work, I'm still glad that we tried. Just being in the study gave me new hope."

Even though Pete was only 25, the MS had destroyed his motor pathways so severely that any hope for recovery was lost. We know this today, that severely disabled people receive little or no benefit from immune suppressive therapy for MS, but at the time we were flying blind.

When the results of our study were published, they were met with a typhoon of controversy. There were too few patients, some said, and those who received placebo worsened much more than would be expected, making our cyclophosphamide-treated group look good by comparison. A later study in advanced MS concluded that nobody in either the cyclophosphamide or placebo group changed very much. But many other physicians who began using the drug for patients like those we studied found that cyclophosphamide helped slow the worsening of MS. The controversy would rage on for more than a decade, and it would take a new technology—the MRI scan—to finally prove that cyclophosphamide did indeed turn off brain inflammation in MS.

Although the benefits of cyclophosphamide were not durable, the experiment was a huge scientific success. We proved the crucial point that suppressing the immune system could stop MS for a time. Now we hoped to build on what we'd learned. Cyclophosphamide was a howitzer, a nondiscriminating DNA poison that destroyed all active cells in its vicinity. We needed something safer that specifically blocked the MS mechanism.

CHAPTER 24

Time in Paradise

Elizabeth and I were married in 1983 by the lighthouse in Owl's Head, Maine, on the first sunny spring Saturday when we weren't on duty, with a justice of the peace who we'd met in a bar the night before. Two college kids walking on the beach below agreed to be witnesses.

Our time as trainees was also coming to an end. I loved Boston, but Elizabeth abhorred the dreary New England winters. She missed the sun and surf of her native California. But we both loved Paris. So, armed with a new round of fellowships, mine in neuroscience and hers in cancer biology, we took off to see the world and sow some oats, more than content to have a few more years as starving trainees before facing real life.

* * *

We planned to run away for a year, but it was Paris, and we were newlyweds, so our escape stretched first to two years, then to three. Fabulous research grants and a historically high exchange rate meant that we could live like royalty, at least by our modest standards. And we couldn't believe our luck when an official at the US Embassy offered us a huge French-classic furnished apartment in the 6th arrondissement near the Luxembourg Gardens.

The lodging also came with a bit of intrigue. The embassy

housing official, a Monsieur Jacques Hadid, rented the apartment to us. It was some sort of side deal, not an official embassy lease. Hadid, a dead ringer for the morally flexible but ultimately kindhearted French constable played by Claude Rains in *Casablanca*, would visit each month to chat and collect the rent—in cash. Once he asked if his daughter could stay in the upstairs maid's room, just for a few months. Of course, we said, and he'd then offer us small favors in return.

The apartment was owned by Mademoiselle Didelot, a dowager who'd retired to Nice. A French aristocrat who still honored America's role in liberating France during World War II, she loved Americans and would only rent to them.

I chose to work at the Pasteur Institute, the oldest and most prestigious biomedical research facility in Europe. I wanted to link immunology with neuroscience, and to my delight, I was welcomed by two superb laboratories, one in each area. Elizabeth found an excellent position at the Hôpital Saint-Louis in the north of the city in a genetics laboratory led by Jean Dausset, who'd won a Nobel for discovery of human transplantation genes, the MHC molecules that immune cells use to communicate with each other.

* * *

I arrived at 8:00 a.m. sharp for my first day of work in the new lab. Nobody was there. Perhaps it was a holiday, or a *grève*, one of those last-minute one-day strikes that are so common in France. I went to a nearby café, coffee and croissant, returning an hour later. Still empty. So I waited in the library. Finally, at about 9:45, a couple of early risers appeared, and by 10:15, the place began to look occupied. Then at 1:00 p.m., everything closed down again. It was lunchtime at the in-house restaurant, three-course meals and rambling conversations. Wine flowed freely. But how could neuroscientists eat sliced lamb brain?

At least there were always baguettes and butter. The lab work would only begin in earnest after lunch and continue through a cocktail hour at 6:00 and often much later. Then a late dinner, and sometimes café hopping that could last hours.

Pasteur was not at all like Harvard.

I was soon anchored in a third laboratory, this one in virology, a nice complement to the ones in immunology and brain science. Each would serve as a building block for my long-term goal to understand MS.

How did a virus lab enter the scene? Just before I arrived, a cataclysmic paper appeared in the journal *Nature*, perhaps the most prestigious journal in science. It was by Robert Gallo, credited as the co-discoverer of the AIDS virus. Gallo reported that he'd found a new virus, closely related to AIDS, as the cause of MS! Maybe Norman Letvin was right—what if MS is caused by a virus and is not autoimmune after all? It was serendipitous that the Pasteur Institute was a world leader in understanding the virus that causes AIDS, and all of the molecular biology tools were at hand to validate and maybe even extend Gallo's findings. I had to jump on this, so I quickly shipped my collection of brain material from Boston to my new lab and drew blood from MS patients I'd begun to see in Paris. With virologist Michel Brahic at Pasteur, I set out to search for the genetic signature of a viral infection in lymphocytes and also brain tissue. It was my first foray back into molecular biology since my days with Khorana at MIT.

There have been many claims of virus discovery in MS, but none stood the test of replication. Almost always scientists would find whatever virus was normally studied in their labs, making the MS claim likely spurious due to contamination. But this time the claim was from Gallo, a giant figure in science. He could not be wrong, I thought. But looking carefully at the paper, I had doubts about the rigor of the work. And using multiple different techniques to detect even minuscule amounts of any virus that resembled AIDS or its relatives, I found nothing, again and again.

So I called Robert Gallo to tell him of my results and ask for his counsel. Where might I have gone wrong? We agreed that the next step should be to convene a small workshop in Washington, DC, where all of the data could be presented and reviewed, and the National MS Society quickly agreed to sponsor the event. I flew back to the United States and met Dr. Gallo in person for the first time. After a couple of background talks by other scientists about human RNA viruses including the AIDS virus, Gallo presented his recently published findings in detail. I followed with a discussion of my negative data, emphasizing that I used several different virus detection methods, including the exact protocol used by the Gallo group. Next was an unexpected presentation, a European group with findings identical to mine.

At the end of the session Gallo raised his hand to speak: "These last two presentations were outstanding. I accept their findings. But I still think that we should continue to search for an MS virus."

As we broke for lunch, Dr. Gallo sought me out. He seemed entirely nonplussed that his discovery, broadcast as front-page news around the globe, had been completely overturned. I was stunned. How could he react to this catastrophic professional setback with such calm equanimity, without an iota of shame?

"I had some doubts about our findings from the beginning," he told me with a smile, "but thought it was important to stir up the MS community to look for viruses."

Earth-shattering conclusions require airtight proof.

* * *

At Pasteur I also learned new ways to manipulate antibodies, the highly specific products of B lymphocytes, and measure their toxicity in autoimmune diseases—practical methods to study immune cells and antibodies and brain cells all together in a test tube.

And for Elizabeth and me, work was not really the main point of it. Our lives were recast, with many new friends, scientists, neighbors, expats, even a few stragglers like us from Harvard. We frequented the symphony and opera, galleries and museums. Visited the countryside and coast. Knew the neighborhood bakeries and charcuteries. Read books and more books. Strolled and wandered. We were young and in love in Paris.

In France, the price of books, music, bread, and other essentials was strictly regulated. Everything sold at list, by law. It kept small businesses afloat, preserving the fabric of local neighborhoods, their idiosyncrasies and quirks. Communities for humans within a giant city. Sometimes rules need to be a little bit intrusive to serve the public good.

Soon we had babies; one beautiful boy, then another. A matronly nanny named Marie-Therese now lived upstairs in the maid's room and became part of the family. (Sorry, Monsieur Hadid, but your daughter will need to move out.) Whenever we spoke English, Marie-T feared we were talking about her, so gradually French became our language not only at work but also at home.

Paradise on Earth.

We almost stayed forever. We had job offers in France, but also in Boston. The turning point was our kids' education, even though it was years away. The French school system was too rigid for my taste. What if our sons behaved as I did? In France, a wild child had little chance for acceptance to an elite school. Youngsters were selected at age 13 or 14 based on ability to sit still eight hours a day, something that nature never intended young boys to do. There seemed little room for late bloomers in France, while second chances existed by the bucketful in the United States.

So we resolved to return home but vowed to carry back with us this newfound lifestyle. When our second child was born at the Hôpital Américain, Elizabeth was served a New Year's Eve feast of wild roast boar garnished with red currants. Aesthetics count. And when we arrived back in Boston, it was the summer of 1986, and we were now a family of four.

CHAPTER 25

Family Life

We'd always have Paris, but after three years of romance, babies, baguettes, and molecular biology, we were back in America.

With help from our families, we cobbled together a down payment for a modest Victorian on a quiet street in the heart of Concord, an easy jog to Minuteman Park, where "by the rude bridge that arched the flood . . . [they] fired the shot heard round the world."* You could almost hear the crackle of the muskets.

Elizabeth and I returned to Mass General, newly minted faculty at Harvard. Elizabeth's position was officially half time, but half time as a pediatric oncologist caring for children with leukemia and other cancers corresponds, more or less, to a full-time job in real life. Reliable childcare would be essential.

Our two Parisian babies, 4 months and 17 months when repatriated, were soon joined by a third, American-born, brother. We were now a family of five. The third floor of our new house could function as an au pair residence, so live-in help was the best solution for our childcare needs. Friends, Mass General docs like us, recommended that we work with an agency on Charles Street in Beacon Hill, near the hospital.

When we arrived for our scheduled appointment, we were

---

* "The Concord Hymn" by Ralph Waldo Emerson.

greeted by an impeccably coiffed and manicured fashionista. "Please tell me about yourself and your style of child-rearing."

"My family is in the boxing business," I answered. "I'd like the boys to be able to defend themselves."

A kick under the table from my wife.

"We both work as physicians at Mass General," Elizabeth explained. "I work part time but need to be at the hospital every day, so it's really important that the person be reliable and very kind. This is what's most important to us."

"All of our child development specialists have degrees in sociology or early childhood education," she replied. "And they all are certified for advanced CPR."

"CPR?" I chimed in. "How often do your child development specialists have to use that on the kids?"

Another kick.

"Do you have any child development specialists with PhDs?" I asked. "We'd really like one with a PhD."

A third kick, this time harder.

"No PhDs at present, but we do have them on occasion," she responded, without a hint of irony. Then turning to my wife, she volunteered, "Elizabeth, we have a couple of superb candidates at the present time. I'm sure that you'll be delighted once you meet them and learn of their qualifications."

Elizabeth now took over. I had failed the interview.

"That sounds wonderful. Could you send us their names and bios? I'd very much like to review those and then call you tomorrow to understand the next steps."

During the first five years we went through 17 nannies in all. The first three were from the agency. Number one hailed from Ireland and seemed lovely, but she had to leave within a few days because she learned she was pregnant. The second, from Nebraska, was immediately homesick and cried nonstop until we took pity on the poor kid and returned her to her family. The third was a young woman from rural Iowa. After a week or so of daily outings to purchase five pounds of flour at a time for constant cookie-baking projects, the boys began looking chubby. We decided it wasn't a good fit.

I lost it. No more live-ins.

But the local options turned out to be no better, even though I could now refer to them as babysitters rather than child development specialists, and we no longer had to transfer our entire salaries to the agency. One disadvantage was that they didn't always show up. An even bigger problem were the remnants of smoking and drinking that we could see, and smell, in our house. And it got even worse.

One day Elizabeth returned home several hours earlier than expected, as her clinic had finished early. It was one of those red-hot, humid August afternoons when the air stuck to your lungs and the clothes to your skin. If she rushed home quickly, there'd be time to take the kids to White Pond to cool off, and maybe then for an ice cream at Kimball Farm in Carlisle, Massachusetts, a picturesque little town just down the road from Concord. She'd spend a few extra hours with the boys and turn a dusty, humid, midweek afternoon into a day to remember.

But the house was empty. No sign of the children or the babysitter, a fiftyish single woman named Yvonne. My wife is a cool customer. Unlike me, she rarely gets frazzled. I always think the worst while she assumes all is well. But not this time. A neighbor had seen Yvonne drive off around lunchtime. A quick search of the library and downtown—the only agreed-upon outings—failed to turn them up. Calls to Yvonne's home went unanswered—this was the era before mobile phones. Ninety minutes later, the longest ninety minutes of her life, as Elizabeth was on phone with the Concord police, Yvonne drove into the driveway. The children were overheated, stuck in their plastic car seats. They were too young to recount what had transpired. Blasé, in a skimpy cocktail dress and high heels, all that Yvonne would say was that she'd visited a friend, and Elizabeth should have told her she'd be back earlier than usual.

The dust soon cleared. Yvonne was kaput, the kids were rehydrated, and they still made it to White Pond for a quick twilight splash. And while all this was going on, I was in the lab, offering moral support by phone but mostly looking at data with a postdoc. When I returned home, it was already dark, the kids were bathed, and dinner was on the table.

It was terribly unfair that this should all be on Elizabeth's shoulders—I had to figure out how to help more. But she told me that whenever I took care of the kids, her work to restore a semblance of order only increased. The kids agreed. Once we were all sledding down Nashawtuc Hill in Concord when our youngest child, who was three, became hungry and cold.

"Mommy, I want to go home," he cried.

"OK, sweetheart, Daddy will take you."

"I don't think Daddy knows how to take care of me," he pleaded, looking up at Elizabeth.

From the mouths of babes.

A tough commute, two demanding jobs, and three in diapers, all at the same time. It was a busy life, and the memories of our days in Paris were fading much too quickly. But somehow, our new life was exhilarating and fun. We had such good times together and were increasingly self-contained. It also worked because we had a secret weapon: Munga.

What really made everything possible was my mom, now retired, now called "Munga" by the boys and soon by everyone else. She was always there for us. We'd call when help was needed, sometimes late at night or at 5:00 a.m.

"Elaine, could you help us?" Elizabeth would ask. The babysitter is ill, or she'd just broken up with her boyfriend and is too depressed to work, or she quit because the kids locked her out of the house. "We need help. Just for the rest of the week, or maybe for about a month, until we find someone new. Can you make it?"

"I have to call my runners' club," she'd answer. "We have a big run tomorrow. I'll tell them I can't join them. And I'll call the Jewish Center to cancel the luncheon today. I can still get my money back. I don't want them to charge me for the meal. I'll leave in half an hour and will be there by 10:00 a.m."

Every time.

Again and again Munga saved us during those busy years. Although she lived in New York, a four-hour drive away, she was as much a part of the lives of our boys as any grandparent could ever be. She was a babysitter, short-order cook, outings director, and a fourth player for two-on-two baseball and soccer games. She'd wheel the kids all around town, three squeezed into a two-seater stroller. And during their naps, she'd mow the lawn. No babysitter or normal grandma could do all this.

CHAPTER 26

Dreams of Genes

Back at Mass General, I was a newly minted assistant professor, and with modest startup funds from my department chairman plus a couple of research grants obtained while still in Paris, the pieces were all in place. Determined to pick up on the MS thread, I opened my own lab, completely independent for the first time, and also created a new clinic for people with MS and other immune diseases of the brain, just as I'd done earlier at the Brigham.

The clinic was as important as the lab. It would allow me to interact with patients, partner with them to find answers, and also teach residents and students, some of whom would also hopefully find inspiration to study MS. I hired a nurse to help me run the clinic, a technician to support the lab, and two postdoctoral fellows whose salaries would be paid by their home institutions. It was lean and mean and terrific.

* * *

During my research fellowships over the previous six years, in Boston and then Paris, I'd learned the basics of immunology and molecular biology. I was determined to apply what I'd learned to study MS, and chose two projects I thought would be key to understanding how the disease develops.

First, I'd use genetics to determine why some people get

MS and why it runs in families and certain ethnic groups. In 1986, the science of DNA analysis was still in its infancy, but it offered the promise of a truly unbiased approach to figuring out the roots of MS. When I studied lymphocyte sensitivity to a brain protein or searched for a specific virus in tissue, I was testing a preconceived hypothesis. But if I could sequence the building blocks of DNA and find changes that were disease related, I would be able to identify the genes and how they work, revealing for the first time what triggers MS. To do this, I'd first need to create libraries of DNA from patients at high genetic risk for MS—those who had several family members with the disease—and use genetic tools to decipher the MS code. Once we found the MS genes, we'd hopefully be able to understand exactly why some people are especially susceptible.

This led to many strange but wonderful road trips, nationwide barnstorming tours for MS research.

Airline tickets and auto rental confirmations in hand, and a large cooler with blood draw supplies fully packed, I traveled to more than 40 states, north, south, east, and west. I'd examine the patients and review medical records to confirm that they indeed had MS, while coworkers would construct family trees and draw blood from affected and unaffected relatives. With help from the MS Society, we created a national hotline for MS patients and developed a center for collection and distribution of genetic samples for researchers around the world. We visited wealthy enclaves, inner-city tenements, suburban towns, isolated mountain cabins, and rural farms. We were invited to picnics and family reunions, often making side trips to nursing homes to visit with relatives too ill to attend. One family had twelve members affected with MS, with others experiencing a plethora of different autoimmune diseases. Another had three affected siblings, now middle aged, living together, helping each other, and hoping that something might result from our work that could benefit their children, several of whom already showed signs of MS. We met a cowboy artist and a palm reader, schoolteachers and high school students, movie stars and priests. Many became my patients.

As our capabilities increased, I was also asked by the MS Society to investigate several reported "outbreaks" of MS: one in a high school class in Loveland, Colorado; another in a group of nurses at a Key West, Florida, hospital; and a third most curious case of a "cursed" house, set on stilts over a pond in rural Maine, where MS developed in three successive tenants. Could we find some clue to the MS trigger here, maybe in the water, or food, or air? Sadly, we could not. The Loveland outbreak was explained by high genetic susceptibility in the community, the Key West cluster in part by hysteria, and the Maine cases by simple misinformation. The sleuthing was exciting, but the conclusions proved mundane.

All of these journeys opened a window into what it means to have MS and to be ill in America. I was especially conscience-stricken to see how difficult it is to have a chronic disabling illness if you are poor and live far from a sophisticated medical hub. I'll never forget the way we were welcomed, fed, and helped in our work by people from all walks of life, who looked to us as their last best hope against a dread disease that had caused such devastation.

One can sometimes learn more from a single trip to a patient's home than a lifetime of clinic visits.

To find the genes that cause MS we'd first need to identify a DNA marker that was related to the disease, meaning a sequence of genetic material that was present more often in affected than unaffected people. But this was only the start. Each marker is located on a "block" about a million DNA bases long, a large chunk of a chromosome, and the true MS change could be anywhere within the block. So even after we identified the general area where a genetic change was present, it would be difficult and maybe impossible to pinpoint the true culprit, the causal mutation. We were searching for a needle in a haystack.

But evolution offered us a powerful shortcut. Our species dates back 180,000 years, approximately 8,000 generations since Adam and Eve. And with each generation our chromosomes scramble, and the blocks of chromosomes that are inherited together get a little bit smaller. When humans first left Africa about 50,000 years ago, only a relatively few of those hearty migrants survived the trip, creating a genetic "bottleneck" where many of the evolutionary adaptations over the previous 130,000 years—mutations, good and bad—were not carried by migrants into Europe and Asia. They remained in Africa, however. The consequences of this bottleneck are remarkable—there is more genetic diversity in any small African village than in all the rest of the world. Moreover, because the history of African populations is older, the blocks of identical DNA are smaller in addition to being more diverse. So if we could find the same MS-related markers in Africans as in whites, we might uncover the genetic cause of MS much more quickly by identifying changes that were common to the blocks from both ancestries.

I thus set out to extend our genetic studies to African populations. Using the same national program that had proven so successful for patients with white ancestry, I now focused our efforts on African Americans with MS. MS is not only prevalent among African Americans, but African Americans with MS do less well than whites; they are more likely to become severely disabled. Maybe we could understand why this was so. Given the importance of the problem, I was hopeful that many in the African American community would wish to partner with us in our research.

We reached out as best we could, visiting African American support groups and National MS Society branches located in areas with large African American populations. We advertised in local newspapers and partnered with physicians and other healthcare professionals who worked in these areas. We were aided by wonderful colleagues in the United States Armed Forces who cared about the mission and helped us identify patients willing to participate. We worked diligently with large teams of coordinators. But by the end of two years we had collected blood samples from fewer than 150 patients, far fewer than would be needed to begin even a small genetic study of MS on African chromosomes. We were stuck. Far too many African Americans were unconnected to the US healthcare system, physically and, even more important, spiritually, and those that we did reach were often fearful of participating in research. Some cited the brutal experiences of Tuskegee and other examples in which African Americans who volunteered for biomedical research had been terribly mistreated. The system that I represented had failed them, time and again, and did not have their trust.

Fortunately, our genetics work was attracting attention, and with the support of several public figures I had opportunities to spread the word through broadcast media. On *Larry King Live*, a talk show on cable TV, I shared a session with Nancy Davis, who'd created an LA-based MS foundation, and Montel Williams. Montel, who spoke movingly about his personal battle with MS, was an immensely popular talk-show host. Moreover, as an African American himself, he enjoyed widespread support within this community. Hearing the importance of African American genetic architecture in solving the MS puzzle, he spoke to me after the show.

"I have an idea. My show has millions of African American viewers. What if you appear on my show and describe to the audience why blood samples from Blacks with MS are so important? I'll share that I'm participating and that everyone listening needs to help us, to help me and many thousands of others. Then you can draw blood from me on TV. Trust me, this will work."

So we did exactly that.

The show aired on a Wednesday. The next morning I walked into the lab to find my lab manager, Robin Lincoln, who'd moved with me from Boston, looking harried and exhausted.

"Dr. Hauser, thank goodness you're here, everything has gone crazy."

"What's the problem?"

"The phones are ringing off the hook. Our answering machine is full, and people have somehow found the main phone into the lab, and your private line also, and they're flooding the hospital with calls asking to participate in our genetics study. And when they can't reach us they just keep calling back, again and again. It's a madhouse."

A tsunami.

We had to act fast. Within an hour we'd contracted with an answering service that could answer twenty calls at a time. We taught the bevy of operators about MS, the study, and the questionnaires that they'd need to fill out for each enrollee. Robin, along with other lab members, were available day and night to help address difficult or complicated issues. We'd need to review everyone's medical records in detail to be sure that the diagnosis was correct. Equally difficult would be to figure out how to obtain the actual blood samples. Some callers lived nearby, so they'd be easy, we could just drive to their homes, but many more were scattered across North America. By early afternoon, Robin had identified a phlebotomy service able to make home visits to draw blood regardless of where patients lived, and we soon had control of the situation. We received nearly 3,000 calls over the next 72 hours.

It would take several years to complete the African American DNA collection. Thanks to Montel Williams, we were able to complete the genetics library required for success. To this day, I'm amazed by his generosity, and also his reach. He'd earned the trust of the community, and was willing to share this precious gift with us.

* * *

The many thousands of DNA samples that we collected formed dictionaries of life that would be used for the next 30 years to decipher the full roster of genes that produce MS risk. Over time, our DNA library was enriched not only with samples from white Europeans and African Americans but also with other populations from around the globe. We collected blood from patients from Japan and China, and on one trip sampled every affected person living in the Republic of San Marino, all providing new opportunities to study different flavors of the DNA blocks that we knew harbored MS genes. And in a series of trans-racial studies we identified a distinctive flavor of a key gene, a master regulator of the immune system, that was inherited uniquely by African Americans with MS, permitting us to decipher the most important genetic culprit in MS and begin to understand how genetics could explain why MS behaves differently in people with certain ethnic backgrounds.*

Technological advances for the study of DNA have been nearly miraculous. In the early 1990s approximately 300 genetic markers were available to search for differences between

---

* Jorge Oksenberg led the early genetic studies in African Americans, and later the partnership expanded with colleagues at Harvard and in particular with David Reich and David Hafler.

individuals; a decade later the number of markers had grown to over a million, and today all three billion DNA building blocks can routinely be identified in any sample, quickly and at low cost.* Most MS risk genes appear to work by regulating how immune cells, and B cells in particular, function.† The unexpected role of B cells identified in these genetic studies would plant the seed for an entirely new approach to treating MS.

This work was exhilarating both because of the patients we met and the promise it held. Now it was time to begin the second project, developing a new model for MS along the lines of what Ray Adams had suggested a decade earlier, one that would accurately reproduce the pattern of brain injury that was wreaking havoc in my patients.

---

* When we published the first full DNA sequence of several people with MS in 2009, the cost was nearly $1 million per person; a decade later this was reduced to less than $1,000.

† This effort would later merge with those of other like-minded initiatives, led by my friends Alastair Compston at the University of Cambridge UK and David Hafler at Harvard and then Yale. We named our global partnership the International Multiple Sclerosis Genetics Consortium (IMSGC). During the past quarter century, the IMSGC has identified more than 230 genetic variants that underlie susceptibility to MS.

CHAPTER 27

A Breakthrough

It was no surprise that Norman Letvin's career had taken off. Less than three years after being banished to the New England Primate Center, a leafy green campus just outside of Worcester, Massachusetts, he'd already become head of immunology at the center. Intense, brilliant, and incredibly focused as always, Norman was close to identifying the virus that was wreaking havoc on the primate colony in Worcester, a discovery that would advance the fight against human AIDS.

Our earlier work on EAE in mice convinced me that the model was useful in understanding how brain inflammation developed, but it taught us little, if anything at all, about MS. Now, several years later, Norman's new role might make it possible to test Adams's idea that MS could be studied more effectively in primates.

It was fabulous to see him again after more than three years, and I remember my excitement as I toured the facilities of the Primate Center, which seemed like a private zoo. I'd always loved animals but needed to keep my distance lest they incite the asthma attacks that had plagued me since childhood. I could handle mice only by wearing a military-grade air mask. As a resident, I had a great, short-lived gig at the local Boston Zoo, where I'd assist the veterinarians with neurologic problems in the animals. The asthma would kick up, but it was worth it.

Among my patients were an epileptic llama and a tiger with colitis and imbalance.

The primate facility was a different experience. No wheezing, not even a sniffle. Even the most allergic among us have no sniffles, no wheezes with monkeys. Their DNA is nearly 99 percent identical to ours, not enough of a difference to be recognized as foreign by our immune system. Allergic to them, you might also be allergic to other primates—like humans.

Norman was studying a beautiful little primate from the mountains of South America, the Callithrix jacchus marmoset.* Adults weigh less than one pound, about the size of a small hamster. And the immune system of these animals is flat-out amazing. Callithrix develop as twins or triplets mostly, and in utero their bloodstreams connect. Immune cells mix, and the embryo learns to recognize the cells of its twins as its own. And throughout life, the immune system of each animal is a mixture of its own cells and those of its siblings. They are chimeras. And because the siblings' cells are present in each animal's body early in life, this should result in deletion of lymphocytes capable of attacking substances on the siblings' cells. Their immune system would be "tolerant"—no longer reactive—to the cells of their brothers and sisters. Norman and I reasoned that this curious quirk of nature should make it possible to transplant cells from one animal to its sibling without causing rejection.†

The implications were stunning.

The advance that launched the modern era of immunology was the development of inbred mice. Take a male and female mouse from the same lakeside community, put them together in a cage, and they fall in love and have babies. And if the babies make babies with each other, and the grandkids do as well,

---

* "Callithrix" is derived from the Greek for "beautiful hair."

† Peter Medawar had won the Nobel Prize for his immune studies with chimeric cows.

and on and on, after twenty or so generations, all of the mice are like identical twins. Genetically identical mice—strains, in the jargon of science—could now be shipped to laboratories around the world, meaning that a scientist in Des Moines studying a strain A mouse should now have the same results as another in Tokyo.*

Using inbred mice, it was also possible to isolate different parts of the immune system from "donor" mice and transplant these, in various combinations, to genetically identical "recipients" that accept the new parts as their own. It's like taking a Ford Thunderbird apart and putting it back together with parts from another identical Thunderbird; Corvette parts don't fit, but Thunderbird parts work just fine. With inbred mice, the role of each cell, each module, of the immune system and how the parts work together could be deciphered. This is exactly what we had done earlier to show that T cells cause EAE, the autoimmune brain disease in mice.

So all of the sophisticated mouse immunology carried out every day in labs all over the medical school could now be applied to Callithrix, and maybe we'd be able to tease apart the immune system in a species that was much closer to humans. This was the chance to test if a true model for MS could be developed in a primate.

I still had concerns about working with monkeys. It helped that these animals are tiny and low on the scale of primate evolution, but they are still primates with complex behaviors and nervous systems. They can feel pain; so can mice and even worms, but monkeys are more likely to feel human-like pain. So I'd do everything possible to minimize any discomfort and use as few animals as possible to obtain valid results. I'd also

---

* An exception is when different bacteria colonize the gut of mice, altering the activity of the immune system.

changed over the years, having seen too many people like Andrea, with terrible MS and no prospects for relief on the horizon. I valued their health more than that of the creatures in the animal colony. When all was said and done, I'd side with my own species.

In those early days, we had extremely ambitious goals but precious little preliminary data. Because we were just beginning a new area of study, we were far more likely to fail than succeed. And this, in turn, meant that there was no way that the project would have received financial support from the federal government. This was true not only for the immunology program, but for the genetics work as well. Thank heaven that the National Multiple Sclerosis Society was there with us from day one, supporting our salaries and the early high-risk experiments. They provided not only funding but also encouragement and moral support, so important for scientists who are just starting out. They shared our passion for the mission to get to the heart of MS.

* * *

We began by testing a variety of different immunization methods on elderly Callithrix,* using animals that had previously been subjects in other scientists' experiments. This involved injecting, just under the skin, small amounts of myelin proteins mixed with different immune stimulants. Each day we'd return to the colony to examine the animals for signs of neurologic disease. Since it was now 1986, we'd also be able to visualize myelin damage with the newly developed MRI technology. Our goal was to see if a neurologic disorder resembling MS would result, something that we'd never seen in mice. Confident that

* We tested the effects of injecting whole myelin, isolated myelin proteins, synthetically synthesized fragments of myelin proteins, and a variety of immune boosters known as adjuvants.

this would happen, at the same time I was also at work testing the immune methods that we'd need to dissect the cause of the MS-like disease that I expected to see. This meant developing reagents that could bind to T cells, B cells, and antibodies from Callithrix so we could measure, isolate, and separately test each of these components of the immune system. We worked hard at it for three years, varying the immunization methods but never producing any disease in Callithrix. Nothing—nada. We could easily reproduce EAE in larger monkeys, as Adams had taught, but Callithrix seemed to be entirely resistant. And only Callithrix were chimeric; sophisticated immune manipulations were not possible in other monkey species. I was frustrated and nearly ready to give up. In science, as in all walks of life, one has to know when to cut bait.

But then the first breakthrough happened. It began with the arrival of a new postdoctoral fellow from Florence, Italy, Luca Massacesi, who would take over the project from a departing fellow. Although he had received a grant from the Italian MS Society specifically to study Callithrix, I now thought that the likelihood of failure was too high. A young scientist has just a few years to make a meaningful contribution, a finding that announces the emergence of a new talent, a rookie soon to be an all-star. Postdocs like Luca need a signature discovery by the time they leave the nest, and mentors have a responsibility to ensure that each young person under their wing departs with an important scientific story to tell.

Luca was just becoming acclimatized to the lab—meeting the team, learning to use the equipment—when I sat him down to tell him of my concerns about the Callithrix project. I expressed disappointment that the fellow he was replacing, a young neurologist, would be returning home with a few modest discoveries but no real breakthrough. I owed it to him, and also to his mentor, a friend who had trusted his most promising young neurologist to my tutelage, to provide him with a better opportunity to succeed.

Luca looked crestfallen, but then eyed me defiantly.

"Steve, listen, please, I've seen your fellow work," he said. "He's afraid of the animals, I'm sorry to say, afraid of the project. Please, I have an idea for a different immunization that might work. Give me three weeks. Just three weeks. I beg you. If it doesn't work, I'll move on as you suggest."

It was true that the departing fellow had a terrible fear of catching an infection from the marmosets. He'd wear three gowns, triple-glove, and heavily tape all potential openings in his armor before going anywhere near the animal facility; he wore face masks everywhere. The procedures required not only technical competence but also passion, and in retrospect I should have seen that his fear meant that his heart was not in the work. Young scientists need to bring new ideas to the table, something that did not happen in his case.

Luca's idea was to try a more powerful type of immune stimulant to boost the intensity of the immune attack against myelin. With luck, this might create the MS-like disease that had eluded us thus far. I gave him the green light: "OK, let's give it a try."

Early on a Monday morning, a few weeks after the immunizations, I received a call from the attending veterinarian to look at two animals who were exhibiting "strange" behavior. Luca and I ran over to the animal facility, huffing and puffing as we changed into the sterile dressing gowns required for entry.

Words were unnecessary—this was a moment that we'd both remember for the rest of our lives.

As experienced neurologists, we could laser in on the changes that the vets had observed. The two animals had developed definite signs of neurologic disease. By this time I'd learned to perform detailed exams on these little animals, but never before had I seen any convincing findings. Today was different. One was leaning against the side of the cage and had grabbed the mesh wall with its left hand. When I opened the fist to release its grip, the animal leaned further to the side, nearly toppling, a clear sign of loss of equilibrium. I held a slice of banana in his line of sight. He grabbed it smoothly with the right hand, but when forced to use the left, a clear upper limb tremor was present. This loss of coordination on the left side of the body signified a disturbance of the cerebellar pathway in the brain, a common feature of demyelination . . . and MS. The second marmoset appeared healthy at first glance, with normal power, sensation, and coordination, but when carefully examined the eyes were crossed, signifying a disruption in the pathway that carries out coordinated eye movements. This indicated a disturbance in the brain stem, the region that coordinates movements of the face and eyes. In humans, brain stem lesions such as this almost always indicate MS—they only rarely occur with other conditions.

Although we'd order MRI scans to confirm our initial impressions, we knew these were MS-like findings. Both animals recovered within a few days, but several weeks later, each developed new and different signs of brain inflammation, loss of sensation, or weakness, only to recover again until the next unpredictable attack occurred. And down the road, after many months, the attacks seemed to stop entirely, replaced by a slowly progressive paralysis.

MRI scans, as we expected, revealed multiple areas of inflammation in the myelin-rich portions of the brain and spinal cord. And when we looked at fragments of brain tissue under a microscope, we saw that the myelin fibers surrounding the tendrils of nerve cells* that reach out to connect with other

* I.e., axons.

parts of the brain were completely destroyed, and the morsels re-formed as bubbles all around the nerves, like the top of a malted milkshake. I'd been searching for this change for more than a decade, and finally, here it was.

I told Luca that he was responsible for this discovery; it never would have happened without his insight and determination. Its importance would grow over time, and it was likely to be the most important advance he'd ever make. We met with the vets and animal handlers to share the results and explain how significant this was for people with MS. We purchased cupcakes for the animals, their favorite food. And we celebrated with our families, a Sunday dinner at Luca's apartment in the Back Bay, meatballs and pasta Florentine style.

I next went to see Edward Peirson Richardson, one of the giants in neurology at Mass General. Dr. Richardson came from the highest rungs of Boston Brahmin society, the blood in his veins carrying the genes of ancestors who had founded the medical school, and the nation. He was a silent philanthropist who kept the entire department afloat each year, all while mentoring generations of young neuroscientists. To us, he was a hero, no less so than his brother Elliot, who, as US attorney general, refused President Nixon's order to fire the Watergate prosecutor, precipitating the Saturday Night Massacre and the end of Nixon's reign.

Dr. Richardson knew as much about the tissue changes that happen in MS as anyone alive. His office was just down the hall from my lab, walls decorated with images from the history of pathology, the centerpiece a handwritten note and image of nerve cells and myelin drawn by Ramón y Cajal, the father of modern neuroanatomy. As usual, I found him stooped over a multiheaded microscope on his desk staring at slides of brain tissue. Button-down shirt, knotted tie, starched short white coat bearing the words "Edward P. Richardson MD, Neuropathology

Service, Massachusetts General Hospital." As I entered the office, he looked up and greeted me in his usual warm manner: "Stephen, how wonderful to see you!"

"Dr. Richardson, can I show you a biopsy from a patient of mine? What do you think is going on?"

He examined the sample in the same slow, methodical way I'd seen him do hundreds of times. First, he raised the slide, with the thinnest possible slice of brain tissue glued to it, so thin that even after staining the proteins and fat with colored dyes, it was translucent. He held it to the light, gently rotated it, looked and looked and looked again, cleaned off a few specs of lint with a fine cloth, examined it again close to the lightbulb, then placed the slide underneath the multiheaded microscope and began to survey the tissue.

"My goodness, this is fascinating," he murmured.

I don't think that in nearly 15 years we ever looked at a sample together that he didn't think was fascinating.

"Really quite remarkable," he continued. "One sees several areas within the section that are clearly demyelinating. Some are acute lesions. Look, here are changes of vesicular demyelination, quite active with a large number of inflammatory cells, mostly lymphocytes and some plasma cells. And here are a couple of areas that are older. You can see the scarring, the plaques; this tells us that the damage is more than two weeks old, but here there is still also active inflammation. And look here, in these lesions, the myelin is completely absent, and the edges separating the plaques from adjacent normal myelin are sharply demarcated. These changes indicate multiple sclerosis, without question. There can be no other explanation."

"Dr. Richardson," I said, "I have to tell you something. This is not tissue from one of my MS patients; it is from a small nonhuman primate with EAE. I'm sorry to have misled you."

A look of astonishment—eyebrows raised, mouth agape.

"No! Really?" he exclaimed. "This is fantastic! Let's compare this to a couple of recent cases."

The similarities were astounding: a perfect replica.

Eliza Doolittle, flower girl judged a princess at the Embassy Ball. Henry Higgins had fooled the experts.

This was the first eureka moment. We now had an ideal model for deciphering MS.

CHAPTER 28

The Left Coast

Joe Martin, my chief at Massachusetts General Hospital, left Harvard around this time—in 1989—to become dean of the School of Medicine at UCSF, the University of California, San Francisco. Soon after, he called me from San Francisco.

"Steve, I'd like for you to visit. You know that the chair of the neurology department here has been open for some time, and I'd like you to look at the department, present a seminar of your work to the faculty, and meet with the members of the search committee. Let's see if this position might be a good fit for you."

"Joe," I replied," I'm flattered to be considered, but I don't think I can move. I'm just getting going at Mass General, and we're well settled in with the boys."

"Please come, just to visit," he said. "No expectations. I've spoken with the chair of pediatrics, and he'd like to meet Elizabeth. There might be a good opportunity here for her also."

I had zero interest in moving. I loved New England and Harvard. To my surprise, Elizabeth agreed with me—she'd done a 180 and no longer yearned to return to northern California despite the lure of her family, the weather, and the Pacific Ocean. Our home was now Concord, Massachusetts.

But I went anyway, just for a visit. And UCSF rocked. It had a dynamism that I've never seen before. The basic scientists and clinicians were all huddled together in tight quarters, sharing closets but also ideas. The Department of Neurology was spectacular, already one of the top three or four in the country. And there was an optimism that it would only get better.

I was only five years out of training, not as well-known or accomplished as any of a dozen neurologists in the department at UCSF. But I hit it off with nearly everyone, save for a few exceptions.

One senior professor asked me if I wanted the job, and I told him I wasn't sure. He responded: "My God, if we can't even get someone like you, we're in much bigger trouble than I thought."

Another was insulted when I told him that he was an inspiring clinician.

"That's code," he said, misinterpreting my comment as a crack against the quality of his lab research. "I see they've gotten to you already." The rift would never heal.

The job had been vacant for a couple of years. The faculty were full of hard drivers with big reputations. But by this time I also had a résumé; although the Callithrix discovery had not yet permeated the field (some things take time), my work with cyclophosphamide, the AIDS virus study, and even my recent report of an immune gene that increases MS risk—my first advance in genetics—had attracted notice. Still, I'd been warned by friends at Harvard that the UCSF crowd would eat me alive. While this didn't concern me, I had little interest in a desk job, or in being a manager.

I told Joe I'd thought it over, but it just wasn't right for us.

He replied, "Steve, let's meet at a little bar called the Stars and Surf, just a block away from your hotel. We can have a drink and can talk it over."

Elizabeth awoke at 2:00 a.m. and saw I hadn't returned. Her instincts told her that the game had changed.

Joe and the school had decided that they wanted us and

wouldn't let any obstacle get in the way. It was a full-court press. They showed us a town in central Marin County built in the 19th century as a summer escape for wealthy San Franciscans that was used to make movies set in New England. They found a way to help us purchase a house in this impossibly unaffordable place, with its quiet streets, excellent schools, mountains and lakes and baseball fields. The animal colony could be moved so that my work could continue, and the key members of my lab were excited about moving with me on an adventure to the West Coast. And the dean reassured me that my main job as chair was to walk the walk as a physician-scientist, as I'd been doing, but also to bring exciting new faculty to the department. This I knew how to do. The management could be done by others.

One of my newfound friends in the department was Stanley Prusiner, who would go on to win a Nobel Prize for the discovery of prions—clumped proteins that hold the secret for brain degeneration. Stan advised me to come but only stay on as chair for five years, after which I could step down and attend to the more important things—the science and the patients.

* * *

Our kids, four, six, and seven years old, got a baseball field in their front yard, and the school was beyond welcoming. Each new child was assigned a buddy, and new families were adopted by neighbors.

Elizabeth is very sociable and high energy, and also inherited a taste for politics from her forebears. She quickly made new friends and was soon running for office, first the school board, then town council, and then mayor, all victories. I also acclimated easily. Most of my friends outside of work were the guys I played basketball with; I was soon ensconced in an even better league in my new town.

Best of all, the asthma that had plagued me all of my life—in New Orleans, New York, and Boston—just disappeared. The children's frequent asthma attacks also melted away. Completely.

Why would asthma go into hibernation? Asthma is as common in the Bay Area as in the suburbs of Boston. To me, this was a powerful lesson in the importance of early life exposures to specific triggers—mold and pollen and germs—that stimulate the developing immune system in early life to provoke asthma. These are different in different regions of the world. Maybe as a child my immune system learned to become allergic to New Orleans or New York varieties, and our kids' immune systems to Paris or Boston ones, but none of us seemed allergic to those in the Bay Area ecosystem. To this day, when a parent with a child suffering from an intractable allergic or autoimmune problem asks me what they should do, I advise them to consider a move to a different part of the country.

I now had more professional responsibilities, but also found that the new position created superb opportunities to accelerate my research. I led one of the elite academic departments of neurology in the nation. I'd reached a new level of visibility, and a large crop of exciting young people lined up to study in my lab. My work could now proceed more effectively and efficiently. I interacted with industry leaders, broadened my perspective, and met new funders, foundations, and philanthropists who wanted to help neuroscience and support MS research. The work quickly moved into a new gear.

CHAPTER 29

Revelation at Sea

The model that we created in Callithrix had all of the hallmarks of human MS. But now that we'd made a model, an imitation, we needed to prove its value as the real thing. It needed to teach us about MS, not just impersonate it. Norman and I had spent nearly a decade developing the experimental toolbox that we'd need to crack the case. We knew how to separate and grow all component parts of the immune system of Callithrix in test tubes, then transplant these into siblings that would accept the donor cells as their own. And we were still confident that autoimmune T cells were the culprits, meaning that T cells, and only T cells, would transfer the disease that we'd created.*

Autoimmune T cells that attack myelin were responsible for EAE in mice.† Take a strain of mouse, any strain, and immunize it with a protein from myelin. Almost any myelin protein will do—take your pick. T cells are always the bad guys. They set off the inflammation in the brain that causes the paralysis and other signs of disease resembling MS. This can be easily proven: just withdraw T cells from the mice sick with EAE, transplant them into healthy, unimmunized littermates, and—bingo—the

* As we've seen earlier, lymphocytes come in different families, and the most prevalent are the T lymphocytes.

† Years later, improved mouse EAE models would be developed that more accurately reflect the immune changes present in human MS.

recipients develop EAE also. Case closed. T cells cause EAE, so they must cause MS as well. Or so most everyone in the field had thought.

A cottage industry formed around pinpointing, with ever-increasing accuracy, the exact T cells (as noted earlier, there are roughly 100 million different kinds [clones]) that produce damage in each mouse model. EAE was the gift that kept on giving: a fertile field for advancing basic science, an engine for publishing manuscripts, and a perfect training ground for young scientists.

For more than three decades, every EAE application for funding began by stating how the proposed work will help people with MS. EAE was MS in a little cage. Sometimes it wasn't even clear if an experiment was being proposed in people with MS or mice with EAE. Even when treatments that worked so well in the mice, and especially treatments that kill T cells, didn't work at all in MS patients, it did little to change the thinking. Humans pivot slowly.

I also drank the Kool-Aid. I thought that T cells were the sole actors in MS and that mouse EAE looked different from the human disease only because the species are so far apart. If we could just test an animal phylogenetically closer to humans, then we'd see that T cells produce demyelination. Now, with the monkey model, this experiment was finally possible. So, we obtained T cells from a Callithrix marmoset with EAE and injected the T cells into its healthy sibling, expecting to transfer the MS-like disease.

We failed, again and again and again. T cell injections never produced the myelin damage that we'd seen repeatedly from Luca's earlier experiments, in which he immunized marmosets with myelin proteins injected under the skin. Our T cell transfers could produce brain inflammation in the marmosets just like in mice with EAE, so they were doing something, but there was never any evidence of exploding myelin, the hallmark of MS. In fact, there was almost no myelin damage at all from the transferred T cells.

Something was wrong with our conceptual framework. Clearly, T cells were unable to produce tissue changes that even remotely mimicked MS, yet the entire world considered MS a T cell–mediated disease. We needed to find the missing ingredient.

* * *

At the end of two years in the laboratory, Luca returned to Florence, turning the project over to Claude Genain, a similarly tenacious young neurologist who had emigrated from Paris.

By this time, I'd shifted the focus away from myelin basic protein (MBP), the protein that had been extensively studied in mouse EAE, to a newly discovered myelin protein named myelin oligodendrocyte glycoprotein (MOG). When we immunized Callithrix monkeys with just a small fragment of MOG injected under the skin, the explosive MS-like myelin changes appeared as readily as they did in Luca's earlier experiments. Could an autoimmune reaction against MOG be the cause of MS? It seemed plausible because MOG is only present in the brain and spinal cord, areas affected in MS, and is completely absent in the peripheral nerves, which are never affected. MOG is located in exactly the same places where MS is found.

Claude began by preparing T cell clones, which is to say batches of identical T lymphocytes, all of which reacted against the MOG protein. We thought that T cell clones would be far more potent in transferring disease compared with the mixtures of different T cells that Luca had used. T cell clones were supercharged attackers. But each time Claude injected the clones into Callithrix, the result was the same—brain inflammation, but never exploding myelin. Never MS-like changes. Exactly what Luca had found earlier with the mixtures of T cells. The transfer of T cells, whether clones or mixtures, never produced the distinctive, groundbreaking pathology that occurred each time we immunized Callithrix with whole myelin or with purified MOG. We were flummoxed.

Sometimes it takes a change of scenery to get a different perspective on your work. Ours came on a motorboat. I hate boats. No matter the size, I feel confined; I abhor the back-and-forth rocking, and I don't like wet shoes. But I needed to get to an immunology meeting on Victoria Island, and so one afternoon Claude and I sat on the bow of a boat together. The scenery must have been beautiful, but we paid no attention, absorbed as we were in trying to decipher the mystery. Why didn't the T cell injections damage myelin? What could we have been missing?

"Maybe antibodies are needed," Claude said.

Antibodies. Maybe it's antibodies and the cells that manufacture them, the B cells. Maybe that's it. B cells and antibodies.

* * *

As we've seen, B cells are a second family of lymphocytes, educated in the bone marrow, and mature B cells produce highly specific chemical bullets known as antibodies. Immediately I thought of old experiments with guinea pigs, back in the 1960s, showing that demyelination in the eye could be caused by antibodies.

One week later and back in the lab, we transferred antibodies from the serum of marmosets along with their T cells. Wow! The myelin exploded and MS lesions appeared. When we tried transferring antibodies alone, nothing—the animals developed no disease. It seemed that full-blown disease required antibodies and T cells together. Perhaps the autoimmune T cells were needed to disrupt the tight blood-brain barrier, which normally prevents toxins and most bloodstream proteins, including antibodies, from entering the nervous system. Once the T cells opened the gates of the brain, myelin-destroying antibodies entered and the disease appeared. Here, we concluded, might lie the secret to MS.

I called Cedric Raine, a colleague who worked at Albert Einstein College of Medicine in New York. Ced was by now the most prominent MS pathologist in the United States.* A spunky, irreverent Welshman with a sharp tongue, he once famously decked his mentor at a medical gathering over a scientific argument.

I told Ced about our findings and asked if he could help us examine the brain tissue from our animals using highly sensitive probes that he'd developed. He offered to fly across the country to prepare and analyze tissues from Callithrix, an investigation that he'd continue to pursue over subsequent months after returning to the Bronx.

From the moment he arrived, Ced went to work, not only studying our marmoset tissue but also comparing the findings with samples that he'd meticulously collected from autopsies of human MS patients.

He was excited to see our model at close hand and agreed that the changes were indistinguishable from human MS. Ced then performed intricate immune studies on the tissue samples and found, in both our model and in human MS, that antibodies were stuck to the surface of the exploding myelin membranes, activating the cluster of proteins known as complement that destroyed the tissue. In Callithrix, the antibodies were bound only to MOG, the myelin protein that we'd used to immunize them. However, in human MS, although a few antibodies targeted MOG, most were consorting with a variety of other proteins in the myelin tissue. In Callithrix, we'd created

---

* By now E.P. Richardson had retired.

an autoimmune response against just a single myelin protein, but in patients with MS, the tissue-damaging immune response was much wider.

We had learned something quite profound about the fundamental cause of MS—that B cells and the antibodies they produce were at the center of the disease process. That was exhilarating. But despite our enthusiasm for the new model, it was still not human MS. And developing a treatment for MS based on the science that we uncovered was now an even more daunting task. Neutralizing the immune response against any single component of myelin would not be enough. We would need a broader blockade. People with MS had become allergic to their entire myelin membrane.*

* Here I use the word "allergic" interchangeably with "autoimmune." Technically, these are not the same, as "allergy" refers to an exogenous substance, usually harmless, that evokes an unpleasant immune reaction, whereas "autoimmunity" implies a disease-producing immune attack against a healthy tissue in the body. However, as we've seen earlier, the words have been used interchangeably in the past, and I've taken literary license and used the designations interchangeably. I trust that my immunology colleagues will forgive this minor transgression.

CHAPTER 30

More Motivation

A Sunday morning call. Charlie Wilson, our chief of neurosurgery and one of the Bay Area's most admired citizens, needed a favor.* Could I see his friend, a young woman who'd just suffered a neurologic catastrophe, maybe a stroke, maybe MS, maybe something else?

Of course I could.

Katherine was an academic and a national advocate for children's health. She met her husband Ethan when both were students at a top-tier law school. They had two adorable young boys. She'd dedicated her life to improving opportunities for people with disabilities, never imagining that she'd soon join this group.

She'd been ill off and on for about 18 months. Her symptoms were unusual, not the kind of thing her docs could get a bead on. Fatigue, dry eyes, dry mouth. Complaints that couldn't be detected with a reflex hammer or a stethoscope. And on a couple of occasions, mildly indistinct vision in one eye or the other. Blood tests were all normal. An eye specialist found inflammation, lymphocytes floating in the liquid of the eye,† and behind,

---

* A Malcolm Gladwell piece in the *New Yorker* (July 26, 1999) was titled "The Physical Genius: What Do Wayne Gretzky, Yo-Yo Ma, and a Brain Surgeon Named Charlie Wilson Have in Common?"

† A condition called uveitis.

in the retina, a few leaky blood vessels* —but not much else. It was a mild autoimmune condition of the eye, benign and easily treated. But there was no answer for her other symptoms.

When she next developed tingling feelings in her hands and feet, her doctor sent her to a neurologist. He examined her, performed a spinal tap, which was normal, and an MRI, which revealed a few abnormal white spots in myelin-rich brain areas.

He'd seen this problem before, the neurologist told Katherine, in young women like her. They were working too hard, pursuing careers when their nature was to be moms. She should have been caring for her two young boys, not giving lectures and serving on blue ribbon panels in Washington, DC. Her neurological exam was perfectly normal. The symptoms were fabricated by her subconscious.

Katherine decided that she would never see a neurologist ever again. Until now.

When I walked into the hospital room, Ethan was standing at her bedside. He spoke for them both, and it was soon clear why. Katherine could no longer speak. She could open and purse her lips, bare her teeth, bunch her eyes, and squish her nose in a failed attempt to communicate, expressions that resembled snarling. Her brain was trying to remember how to speak. But the only vocalizations were a few grunts. And tears, lots of tears.

It had begun 36 hours earlier, Friday evening, just after dinner. She complained of numbness on the right side of her body, from forehead to toes, a mild headache, and a vague sense of imbalance. She was no better on Saturday morning, and gradually Ethan noticed that something was wrong with her speech: subtle at first, but then no question, it became halting, slowed, robotic. Several days earlier she'd complained of

---

* Retinal vasculitis.

dry eyes and blurry vision, symptoms that had also preceded earlier episodes of numbness.

The damage was smack in the middle of the thinking half of the brain, the left hemisphere, in a small area controlling voice production as well as mathematics and orientation capabilities. The language recognition center, located just behind and below, was not damaged, so she understood most everything that was said, but couldn't follow gestures; her writing was reduced to illegible scribbling, and her recognition of numbers was entirely gone. Patients who lose the meaning of language are often unaware of their deficits, but Katherine was in the opposite situation. She knew what was going on but could no longer communicate with the outside world.

It is always more likely that an unusual illness is due to an uncommon form of a common problem, rather than a common form of a rare one. The physicians in the emergency unit suspected that Katherine had suffered a stroke, but stroke is uncommon in healthy young adults. Because of Katherine's earlier symptoms, I was certain that the problem was caused by an inflammation, and likely an unusual form of MS, common in this age group. I explained this to Katherine, Ethan, and the neurosurgeon who by now had joined us, and set in motion a plan to wheel her down to the MRI machine. The radiologist on call agreed to return to the hospital to assist with the urgent scan.

I'd seen this before, a carbon copy, in the sister of a colleague on the East Coast. She had done pretty well, and maybe with some luck, Katherine would too.

But the MRI results indicated that Katherine's problem was much worse. She had a huge ball of inflammation in the myelin-rich tissue of the parietal, or middle, lobe on the left side of the brain, just as I'd suspected. But the unexpected discovery was another mass, nearly as large, in the back of the brain on the right side. Although this ugly lesion was located smack dab in the vision area of her brain, surprisingly it had produced no symptoms, at least not yet. And in addition to these two red-hot, inflamed, swollen areas of damage, there were several others, smaller but also new and also red hot, as well as a few old scars that had once been inflamed sometime in the past. The same scars that her neurologist had attributed to "wanting to have it all."

It was hard to conceal my dismay. If it had just been a single mass, it might not ever return; it would leave a scar, and maybe some permanent neurological damage, but after recovery, she'd be out of the woods. But multiple lesions meant that this would recur down the road. Katherine had MS, and a terrible form of it.

The first step was to extinguish the inflammation as quickly as possible before more brain tissue was destroyed. I recommended that we begin with high doses of steroids, plus plasma exchange to clean the blood by removing antibodies and other damaging proteins. With these treatments, the inflammation often begins to settle down after a few days, but when more than a week passed and Katherine was no better—she was now becoming weak on the right side—I repeated an MRI scan that showed we had made no headway.

So, I went to DEFCON 2, advising a brain biopsy of one of the injured areas to be sure that our diagnosis was correct. This is a frightening procedure for patients, as it involves a neurosurgical operation: a hole is drilled in the skull and a large needle inserted into the depths of the brain, selecting an area that is abnormal on the brain scan but not performing a critical function.* Despite the daunting nature of a brain biopsy, in experienced hands it is

* In medical terms, a non-eloquent region. Regions of the brain that subserve essential functions are known as "eloquent areas."

actually quite safe and can provide lifesaving diagnostic information. In Katherine's case, the biopsy confirmed that there was no infection, no tumor, no stroke, but the findings were otherwise inconclusive because the damage was so extensive that we couldn't see much living tissue at all. We couldn't reconstruct the battlefield because all that we could see was debris, like Guernica after the Nazi bombings. And when she continued to worsen, we went ahead with a second brain biopsy, now of the large mass on the right side in the back. And this time the tissue could be read with more confidence.

There was no doubt. It was MS.

In catastrophic situations like this, it's important to make a correct diagnosis with as much certainty as possible, as early as possible, because it is likely that no one will ever review the problem again with as fresh an eye or in greater detail. A diagnosis stamped with authority by a "name brand" in the field tends to stick, even when it is wrong. Errors made by luminaries are among the most damaging mistakes in medicine.

Slowly, over many weeks, Katherine stabilized and then gradually improved. Her language returned, just as it had with my other patient, always slightly halting and with a Swedish-sounding cadence. And Katherine could now walk, albeit with a limp, travel, and even return to the lecture circuit.

But like most other young people with MS, she continued to have new attacks from time to time. We tried the newly available injectable therapy interferon, which was designed to fight viral infections but probably worked in MS by tamping down the immune system. She soon realized, though, that the benefits were negligible, repeated injections were a pain, and each new shot brought flu-like symptoms. So, like many other patients, she stopped injecting herself.

"What else can I do?" she asked.

I told Katherine of my experience with cyclophosphamide

chemotherapy, that it stopped the march of MS but for most people the benefit was very short-lived, less than a year. And I mentioned that the treatment was also quite toxic: hair loss occurred, and there was a risk of bladder cancer. Desperate to preserve her remaining function, she decided to try it. Unfortunately, it also didn't help much.

Then, after slowly simmering, year after year, MS struck again, massively this time. Her symptoms included persistent hiccups, difficulty swallowing and breathing, and terrible paralysis in the arms and legs. We found another hot ball of inflammation on the MRI scan, but this time in the worst place in the nervous system, a congested space the size of a thumb, where the brain stem connects to the top of the spinal cord and all the nerve fibers from the brain travel down to control the face, arms, legs, and the rest of the body. Similar to Andrea's case, Katherine's MS struck the main crossroad of her nervous system.

And this happened just as I was beginning to understand the implications of my lab work identifying antibodies and B cells as prime actors in MS. The treatment possibilities that might result from the work were still only vaguely germinating in my mind. My progress was too slow, and Katherine became ill too early.

I admire Katherine and Ethan immensely, but I'm always sad when they visit. Sometimes I almost dread seeing them. They come to the clinic with an attendant who helps Katherine with dressing and care, makes sure she is strapped to the wheelchair lest she slump over, assists with sips of water, and suctions secretions to prevent choking. Katherine is now quadriplegic. At her stage of MS, there is very little I can do to help her.

In a recent correspondence, I wrote to her that I wished I could have done more when her MS first appeared—had I only known then what I know now. I admitted that, in a sense, I felt as if I'd failed her.

She wrote me back almost instantly, "Please don't feel this way, or ever say this to me again. It makes me very sad to think that I make you sad. You did everything that you could. I need you as much as ever, even though you can't help my MS."

Sometimes the roles of the patient and physician are reversed.

CHAPTER 31

Birth of a New Technology

IDEC Pharmaceuticals was founded in 1986 on a dream that technology could be used to create a new type of medicine based on a billion years of evolution, a customized antibody, genetically engineered, that would have the capability of highly selective effects on the body. It was the dawn of the biotechnology industry. The small start-up in San Diego would soon be flying high, but not before a few near collapses, free falls with faulty parachutes. It's not easy to start a revolution. Fortunately, Bill Rastetter, my old roommate at MIT, took over as CEO, and through a combination of fearlessness and drive, would ensure that IDEC reached its life-changing potential.

Evolution created an immune system made up of a hundred million different antibody molecules, each one binding, ever so tightly, to just one protrusion on a cell membrane. What if you could make unlimited quantities of a specific antibody of your choosing, a "monoclonal antibody," so called because each molecule is exactly the same, selected to attack a disease-causing culprit, perhaps a cancer or an autoimmune cell?

The idea that evolution could be harnessed to create a new type of medicine was not new—indeed, it was more than a century old. It was the idea behind the first Nobel Prize in Medicine, awarded to Emil von Behring in 1901, who injected diphtheria toxin into horses and harvested their antibody-containing serum from the bloodstream, an "antiserum," to use as immune therapy against diphtheria.

Fast forward 80 years, and antisera technology was about to take off into the stratosphere.

The enabling breakthrough was a method to produce unlimited quantities of monoclonal antibodies. This discovery had won Cambridge University's César Milstein and Georges Köhler the Nobel Prize,* and labs all over the world raced to make use of the new weapon. It would now be possible, for example, to make a monoclonal antibody against any type of blood cell in the body, and by attaching a label to the monoclonal, the cell could be separated and studied as never before. Within a couple of years, Ellis Reinherz, a medical school classmate of mine, developed a group of monoclonal antibodies while working in Stuart Schlossman's lab at Harvard that could identify different types of human T cells, count how many are in a person's blood, and study how each type functions in a test tube.

While all of this was going on, down the hall from Reinherz was another schoolmate of mine, Lee Nadler, also a human immunologist but whose focus was on B cells. These were the days when the action was in T cells, so Lee was less visible, but he'd soon launch a revolution that would change the MS world. In 1980, he made a monoclonal antibody in a mouse that stuck to a protein on B cells, and then infused it into a patient with a B cell cancer, a form of lymphoma and the most common hematologic cancer in adults. This patient's cancer had been resistant to traditional chemotherapy regimens. The cancer still won, but the patient tolerated the

* Milstein, the lab director, was an Argentinian Jew whose parents had emigrated from Ukraine. Köhler, the force behind the discovery, was a graduate student who helped support his family by driving taxis in his spare time.

treatment reasonably well, and, equally important, the infused monoclonal antibody was successful in killing some of the cancerous B cells in the body. This meant that monoclonal antibodies not only bind and kill cells in test tubes but they could also work in living human beings. And the next year, Nadler's group made another monoclonal, one that adhered to a different protein on the surface of B cells that they called B1; it would soon be renamed CD20.

It is now 1984. Michael Jackson's hair catches fire while filming a Pepsi commercial; the Portland Trailblazers select Sam Bowie ahead of Michael Jordan in the NBA draft; and a second new technology is unveiled, a recipe to replace the backbone of any mouse antibody with a human version, leaving the unique "clonal" sequence that targets a specific structure unchanged. Now mostly human and only part mouse, the genetically engineered, *chimeric* antibody would still stick to the same protrusion on the cell membrane, but could work more effectively in a human body while causing less of an allergic reaction against mouse protein. This could be a drug.

The race was on, and IDEC was determined to win it. Bill Rastetter's idea was to make a chimeric monoclonal antibody that would stick to a person's cancerous B cells, killing them while leaving all other cells in the body untouched. His aim was to cure cancer.

IDEC soon began manufacturing monoclonal antibodies against cancerous B cells in patients with advanced B cell lymphomas. In a small preliminary study, the treatment was effective 20 percent of the time. Some patients went into complete remission for six or seven months, results that were previously unobtainable. Others responded to the treatment for shorter periods of time. The trouble was that each B cell tumor was different. This meant that a different drug would need to be individually tailored for each patient. To do this, the cost of treating one patient would be $50,000, a sum beyond anything that was commercially viable at the time.

We still held to the quaint idea that drugs should be affordable. Bankers were the most conservative people in town, and the value of a drug, even a lifesaving one, had a ceiling. Nobody would have guessed that patients, societies, and governments would one day pay millions to improve the health of a single individual as they do today, for example, to treat a paralytic muscle disease in children with a drug that corrects the genetic mutation.*

But back then, IDEC concluded that although the science was intriguing, this was not a commercial opportunity. They needed a better idea, a single therapy that would be effective for all B cell cancers rather than one that had to be custom made for each patient. Finding the right path to a new kind of drug was by no means an easy task. But a path forward had already been charted by Nadler and his crew at Harvard—CD20.

CD20 is a protein that is found on the surface of B cells, both normal and cancerous ones. For several reasons, CD20 proved to be an ideal target for a drug. It's hard-wired on the outer cell membrane and not easily shaken off or ingested, like many other proteins. It just stays on the surface. CD20 is a sitting duck, always there for the drug to find it. Even better, CD20 is present only on some B cells. It's absent on the youngest B cells that live in the bone marrow, and also on the most mature B cells, the best antibody producers called plasma cells. Sparing the youngest B cells, the babies, means that the immune system grows back after treatment. Leaving plasma cell elders untouched means that the body's immune history, all that it has learned over a lifetime to fight off infections, is also intact.

---

* Onasemnogene, trade name Zolgensma, manufactured by Novartis, is used to treat spinal muscular atrophy.

Bottom line—when someone treated with a CD20 antibody becomes infected, say with a flu virus, the immune system can still mount an effective immune response against the invader. One could never have predicted that destroying B cells would turn out to be so safe.

IDEC began the experiments using an early version of the recipe that within a few years high school students would employ for summer projects: Immunize mice against the CD20 protein. Isolate the mouse B cells and mix their DNA with tumor cells, *immortalizing* them so that the mouse B cells can grow forever. Select one immortal B cell that makes antibodies that stick particularly tightly to CD20. Use genetic engineering to replace the backbone of the mouse antibody gene with its human counterpart. Grow cells producing the "chimeric" antibody, part mouse and part human, in stainless steel tanks. Finally, harvest the "drug"—the antibody.

Whew.

The first person they treated in March 1993, a patient with a very high number of malignant lymphoma cells, developed chills and fever during infusion of the antibody. But they learned that by slowing the rate of administration and treating symptoms with antihistamines and acetaminophen, the reaction could be controlled, allowing the patient to receive the full dose. They were on their way.

The company almost went into bankruptcy twice, but within a few years, they achieved what was needed to move forward—convincing, though only preliminary, evidence that the drug could work. At the time, many patients with B cell lymphoma could be expected to live only one to two years from the time of diagnosis, a dismal prognosis. When the new drug was first tested in patients who had failed conventional regimens and would soon die, responses were seen in 50 percent, lasting on average nearly a year. This was an extraordinarily positive signal—they were on the right track. They'd now have enough data to approach a larger company, Genentech, for assistance in carrying out the pivotal phase 3 study, the final trial required to prove the drug's value and safety. A partnership was established in 1995, and the larger study, involving 166 patients, could thus be carried out and would soon confirm the earlier findings.

Two years later, the CD20 antibody rituximab, marketed as Rituxan, received FDA approval for treatment of B cell lymphoma. Its use as standard first-line therapy would help to revolutionize prospects for patients with these cancers, and today more than two-thirds of patients can expect to be cured.

I watched all of this from afar, delighted with my old roommate's success, and was beginning to imagine that—just perhaps—Bill's new drug might also be useful for other B cell problems, not only for cancer. Maybe it could help people with MS.

CHAPTER 32

Struggling for Funding

Physician-scientists work in two worlds. The scientist searches for deep answers, the root cause of disease. The physician cares about this, of course, but is also motivated to do more for suffering patients. And so it was with us. We now knew that B cells and antibodies were incriminated in MS, but we didn't know exactly how, and this would take many more years of work to sort out. It was now possible, however, to think about immediate applications of what we'd learned.

My colleagues and I wrote a grant application to the National Institutes of Health (NIH) requesting funding from the federal government for a clinical study to see if my college roommate's drug, rituximab, which killed B cells, could benefit people with MS.* We worked weekends and nights to make the best possible case and designed a study to efficiently test the merit of this approach. I was cautiously optimistic that funding would be awarded.

Then we waited. And waited and waited. It takes more than six months for an NIH application to be reviewed by a committee of peers, termed a "study section," and for results of the review to be communicated back to the scientists. Even when the

* This grant had been championed by a team that also included Nancy Monson and Michael Racke at the University of Texas Southwestern Medical School, and Claude Genain at UCSF.

review is favorable, it takes more than a year from submission to initial receipt of funding. More often, the committee will be supportive but request a revised application to address their concerns, a process that adds a second year. I was hopeful that the study would be funded, but was also prepared to resubmit if necessary.

The review, when it finally came in, hit like a ton of bricks.

"The concept is biologically implausible," it said.

Our application was rejected. But the feds offered an olive branch. In a call with the director, I was told that if we tabled this B cell nonsense and were willing to test a T cell therapy, they'd consider funding our team.

"Just forget your last 15 years of work, kid, and do what we think you should do."*

I couldn't really blame the NIH. The federal government has to rely on expert referees to guide funding decisions, and experts usually reflect prevailing beliefs. Peer review ensures that fewer crackpots are funded, but high-risk/high-reward science can be a casualty. This outcome dashed our hopes that public funding could ever be mobilized to support the trial. I needed to find another way to fund a treatment study in MS, and quickly, because by now I was confident that rituximab could help people with MS.

How could I have been so confident? Simple—even though rituximab had never been approved for MS, I'd already been using it with several difficult-to-treat patients, people not responding to available MS drugs or unable to tolerate their side effects. I carefully informed each one of the uncertainties and risks of using an untested drug, such as severe infusion reactions, but all enthusiastically agreed to try it. And what they, and I, saw was convincing. Most had no further MS attacks; the

---

* He didn't really say it in this blunt a manner, but this was the basic message.

disease seemed to stop in its tracks. My clinical instincts knew that something very special was happening. I had no proof yet, but these encouraging responses fueled my resolve. Despite what the government experts thought, I was determined to find a way to test rituximab in MS.

CHAPTER 33

Against All Odds

The new millennium arrived with a bang, and it was proving to be a year of failed predictions—our computers didn't crash, and the rapture didn't happen. I was determined to add to the list the NIH's conclusion that B cell therapy wouldn't work in MS. The moment that they rejected my application, I began discussions with Genentech about using rituximab for MS. It was my next best option. Genentech was just a short hop down Highway 101, one of many advantages of living in the Bay Area. The company had extensive relationships with UCSF. Genentech had been co-founded by Herb Boyer, a UCSF faculty member, and the original patent that launched the company was held jointly by UCSF and Stanford. I also had excellent relationships with the scientists at Genentech, including Craig Smith, a neurologist who was also a colleague and friend. Before he joined Genentech, Craig and I had worked together on research in optic neuritis, a form of MS. Craig was a formidable figure. He hailed from Alaska and was a national champion rower whose father, Merle "Mudhole" Smith, was a legendary bush pilot and a founder of Alaska Airlines. Craig immediately understood the potential value of rituximab for MS, and soon I had a powerful advocate at the company.

There were other advantages to working with Genentech. In addition to deep pockets, they had tremendous expertise in carrying out human clinical trials and dealing with the FDA and other regulatory agencies. My cyclophosphamide study had taught me how difficult it was to carry out even a small clinical trial in an academic environment. But it was now 20 years later, and the administrative and regulatory requirements for human research had increased manyfold since then. In these areas, Genentech was a pro. They knew how to perform highly successful clinical trials. On the negative side, by working with industry, I might lose some control over how the trial was conducted and the data would be analyzed, but I was confident that I could navigate any challenges that might arise.

I also learned that the pharmaceutical giant Roche had independently approached IDEC with the idea that rituximab might be useful for the autoimmune joint disease rheumatoid arthritis. They decided to move forward on a trial to test the concept. It was good news for me that Roche was willing to test B cell therapy in rheumatoid arthritis, a disease, like MS, that had been conventionally considered to be T cell-mediated. I was convinced that the rationale for testing rituximab in MS patients was even stronger than for arthritis.

Just as my discussions with Genentech were reaching their final stage, another merger was taking place. IDEC was about to merge with Biogen, an event that would change the landscape for rituximab in MS. Biogen at the time was a successful but one-dimensional enterprise fueled by profits from its beta interferon drug for MS. Interferon didn't work very well. It reduced MS attacks only modestly; signs of new disease continued to appear on MRI scans. Moreover, interferon had no benefit against gradually progressive disability. Biogen was also in the late stages of developing a second MS drug, natalizumab, that worked by blocking a molecule that lymphocytes use to move across blood vessel walls and enter the brain.

From Biogen's perspective, rituximab could become a competitor to their lineup of MS drugs. They now owned rituximab through the merger with IDEC, and it seemed likely (as some speculated) that they wanted to prevent its use for MS. This wasn't illogical. Few believed that it would work anyway, and even if it did, rituximab was inexpensive and would siphon away profits from their more costly MS drugs. But Biogen's hands were tied. IDEC already had a co-development deal with Genentech stipulating that Genentech could move forward on its own for future uses of rituximab. At Genentech, though, outside experts in the MS field were also advising the company not to move forward, and internally, prognosticators—Genentech's Merlins—estimated the chance of an MS trial being successful at less than 15 percent. They agreed with the NIH.

In early 2003, I attended an urgently scheduled meeting at Genentech's headquarters in South San Francisco to present, for the umpteenth time, the arguments for the rituximab trial in MS and respond to the naysayers. After several hours of give-and-take, and hearing all the reasons why his company should not assume this risk, Genentech's leader, Art Levinson, spoke up: "For God's sake, patients need this, badly, and if we can't do this, why are we here in the first place?"

This broke the logjam. And at Biogen, fate was now on our side as well. Rituximab was Bill Rastetter's baby, and my old college roommate had just been named CEO of the newly merged company, Biogen IDEC. You just could not make this up.

There would be other, equally consequential challenges ahead arising from patent and turf wars, but at least we could move forward with a preliminary study to test the idea that B cells cause MS and that a drug that targeted B cells could be effective. And once the program was green-lighted, our planning rapidly moved into the fast lane; within weeks we were ready to enroll the first patient in the study.

* * *

Three years later, the last Friday of August 2006 was one of those spectacular afternoons that grace late summer in Northern California. New England without the bad parts—no need for mosquito spray or umbrellas, and the good weather lasts longer than eight hours. The beginnings of fall appear as leaves turn bright shades of yellow and red. A cool, clean breeze is in the air, but the late afternoon sun is still warm enough for swimming.

It was also a day of hope, for this was the day we would "unblind" the results of our first study treating MS with a B cell antibody. We'd see if the treatment worked.

It was a miracle that we'd made it this far. The cards were stacked against us—most everyone, including the feds, was convinced that the Ts, not Bs, were the perps in MS. B cells were the good guys, they said; kill them off with rituximab and you'll make MS worse. That's what happens in the mice. If our treatment does the same to people, we'd hurt them, maybe even kill someone. First of all, do no harm.

And there was another, far more vexing reason for concern that the clinical trial could fail. Even if we were correct that antibodies, those highly specific immune bullets made by B cells, cause MS, they would not be quickly destroyed by rituximab. This is because when a B cell is activated, it turns into an antibody-producing factory, a big muscular plasma cell that manufactures thousands of bullets each second. And, as we've seen, plasma cells no longer have the CD20 protein on the surface. It's turned off. So, rituximab won't kill them, and we have to wait until the plasma cells die from old age. Which may take years.

In "placebo-controlled" trials, the gold standard for testing new therapies, neither the subjects nor the physicians know who receives the test medicine and who receives a placebo. Our original plan had been to treat 200 patients with one of two treatments—half would receive rituximab, two doses spaced six months apart, and the other half identical-appearing placebo injections. At regular intervals after beginning the trial, brain inflammation would be measured with MRI scans. The level of inflammation at 12 months would be the primary endpoint, or first goal of the study. Other endpoints were the number of MS attacks, changes on the neurologic exam, and safety. It was planned as a phase 2 trial, meaning that it was only preliminary and larger follow-up trials would be needed to be sure that the treatment had clear-cut benefit over the long term.

The MRI scan is much more sensitive than other tests used to detect inflammation, the hallmark of disease activity in MS. Using MRI as the outcome measure meant that we needed fewer patients to see a beneficial effect of a treatment. To approve a new drug for use in MS, however, the regulatory agencies require proof that the treatment improves how patients function. It's not good enough to see an improved brain scan. An effective drug should make people feel better, walk better, see better. These studies, called phase 3 trials, are complicated and expensive, usually involving several thousand, rather than a few hundred, patients. We had proposed as a first step to conduct a preliminary phase 2 study. This would cost Genentech around $60 million, an enormous sum for a laboratory but pocket change for a biopharmaceutical company.

But when we told the FDA of our plan, they balked, concerned that the risks were too great and that patients in our trial would be denied treatments for MS that were currently in use. We were stunned. At the time, there were only two modestly effective therapies available for people with MS. Both required frequent injections and had bothersome side effects. Most patients chose to take nothing. But the feds had told us to cut the size and duration of our study in half. We could enroll only 100 patients, 50 in each group, give only one dose of the drug or placebo, and wrap it up just six months later.

Our prospects for success were even further diminished. Genentech's new estimate of the likelihood of a positive outcome was now less than 10 percent, but somehow Craig and I kept the trial alive. Bolstered by confidence that the drug would work if given a fair chance, I clung to the belief that we'd still see a beneficial effect from this now diminished, inadequate study as I had with my own patients. But could I be wrong? In my lectures describing my new thinking that MS might be a B cell–mediated disease I'd mention the possibility that rituximab could be effective. Several months after a talk at Harvard, my former stomping ground, a colleague who'd heard my talk called.

"We tried rituximab. It doesn't work."

So I had ample reason to worry, despite my confidence in all that I'd learned from the lab and seen at the bedside. The trial was now so reduced in size that maybe a positive effect would be missed. One thing was certain: we'd be given only one shot on goal. There wouldn't be a second chance. But I was also confident that any positive trend, even a hint of some favorable response, could justify a return to the FDA with a request to conduct a more meaningful, longer-term trial.

So needless to say, when we unblinded the trial on that late August afternoon, the stakes were high. A small group of statistical experts had been at work for several weeks "cleaning" the data, making sure that each entry for each patient, from first to last, was complete and accurate.

When we opened the folder containing the results, what we saw was extraordinary: there was a nearly complete, and almost immediate, elimination of inflammation in rituximab-treated patients! And improvement was already evident on the very first MRI scan, taken just four weeks after treatment as a precautionary safety measure added to be sure that by removing B cells we did not make MS worse.* By the next MRI eight weeks later, MRI activity was reduced by more than 90 percent, a positive effect that was sustained throughout the duration of the study. There were also big reductions in new MS attacks, which was amazing because the study was so small. But most stunning was the rapid onset of action. Because the benefit appeared almost immediately, it could not have been due to a reduction in disease-causing antibodies, as this would have taken much longer to occur. The only reasonable explanation was that the B cells themselves were at the heart of MS.

Nature had revealed one of its closely guarded secrets—how the brain was attacked. The program leader at Genentech, Michele Libonati, with whom I'd worked arm in arm, who rode shotgun to make sure we could stay the course despite the obstacles, whose career was on the line with this one, could not contain her tears, a mixture of relief, exhaustion, and joy.

We'd discovered an incredibly potent, effective, and apparently safe new treatment. It was not by accident, but our conceptual framework, our underlying ideas, were also not entirely correct. It worked much faster than predicted. We were correct that B cells were at the center of MS; by knocking them out of the bloodstream, we'd shut down the disease to a degree never before seen. But the benefits could not be due only to removal of B cells producing antibodies, like in Callithrix. In people with MS, antibodies were still important, we were sure of this from our studies of MS brain tissue with Cedric Raine. But antibodies could not fully explain how B cells attacked the brain. This was all more than OK; humbling, but in some ways the best possible outcome, even better than being completely right.

---

* As described earlier, mice with T cell–mediated EAE are worse when B cells are removed.

We could now return to the laboratory to refocus our efforts to understand how B cells, not only through antibodies, misbehave in MS. And most important, we'd identified a treatment likely to help millions of people while learning something completely unexpected about the cause of this disease.

* * *

In accordance with securities law, results of the trial were publicly communicated on the next business day, the following Monday, August 28, 2006. It was a joint communiqué from Genentech and Biogen IDEC. Quotes from the two companies were different in tone, however, reflecting a divergence in outlook and enthusiasm for what we'd accomplished. Biogen was cautious and circumspect, noting that they were "committed to offering multiple options for people with MS." By contrast, Genentech's press release conveyed my enthusiasm, noting that the results "exceeded our expectations" and supported "our hypothesis that B cell targeted therapy may play an important role in the treatment of MS."

I paid little attention to the sound bites, distracted as I was by the magnitude of what we'd accomplished.

CHAPTER 34

Trials and Tribulations

Eight months later, I presented the rituximab results at a global neurology meeting in Boston. This was the first time the scientific community would see the actual data in detail. There was standing room only in the large hall of several thousand. Everything had to be perfect, and it was. All the work had been done in advance, and the data were stunning. And at the end, I was prepared for every possible question, including one big one in particular that came as expected: "At baseline, more patients in the rituximab group had active MS compared with the placebo group. Have you considered the possibility that your results are due to regression to the mean?"

Translation: MS naturally waxes and wanes, and if you enroll patients into a study at the peak of their disease activity, the disease will often quiet down on its own. Rituximab may have had nothing to do with the outcomes.

"The baseline imbalance arose from the relatively small size of the study," I replied. "The differences between the two groups at entry were modest, while the magnitude of the treatment effect was robust. We performed numerous sensitivity analyses to test for possible confounders, and each supported the validity of our conclusions. Minor statistical variations are common in small phase 2 studies."

Translation: the effects of rituximab were so dramatic that

small differences between the rituximab and placebo patients at the time of enrollment were meaningless.

I was confident that our conclusions were correct, but still wished that the FDA hadn't forced us to reduce the size and duration of our study.

On my way out the door I saw my friend from Harvard, the one who called to tell me that rituximab didn't work.

"Rituximab is really amazing," he said. "We've been using it, and it is miraculous. Unbelievable!"

I don't think he remembered his earlier call.

That evening we celebrated together, academic investigators from three continents with our partners at Genentech, an evening of good cheer fueled by enormous hope for the future. It felt as if we were riding a freight train that couldn't be stopped. Rituximab would soon be widely available for people with MS. The prospects for patients were simply too promising to be derailed.

I seriously underestimated the difficulties that lay ahead.

* * *

Large-scale phase 3 clinical trials demonstrating efficacy and safety are the final step before any new drug can be FDA approved* for use in a specific disease. I was confident that these would begin promptly, leading to rapid approval by regulators and delivery to our patients. We targeted 2010 as a reasonable goal to complete the needed studies. Already many MS experts were, like me, beginning to use rituximab off-label for their patients. Physicians are given wide berth in making treatment decisions; half of all US prescriptions are off-label, meaning medications prescribed for conditions not formally approved by regulatory agencies. But this comes with a cost. Once a treat-

---

* Other regulatory agencies, such as the European Medicines Agency (EMA), must also approve the drug before it can be used within their jurisdictions.

ment becomes standard, it's difficult and often impossible to test it against no treatment. In developed countries, physicians and patients aren't willing to accept the possibility of receiving placebo rather than a drug that appears (but is not proven beyond the shadow of a doubt) to be effective, and it's considered unethical to conduct trials only in economically disadvantaged areas of the world where the drug is not otherwise available. And from the company's perspective, why spend the money to formally test if your drug works when it's already in wide use and commercially successful?

So for rituximab, it was critically important to conduct the definitive trials quickly. But with a price tag of $800 million dollars, we were dependent on funding from Genentech. The ball was now entirely in their court.

Another year passed, and still no progress had been made. From Genentech: radio silence. The steady communication that was a hallmark of our relationship had waned, slowed to a trickle, then evaporated. Kaput. Worse yet, my close friends and colleagues at Genentech soon left, each departure accompanied by a public statement about the chance to pursue other opportunities, spend more time with family, and ruminate on their deep gratitude to the company. Orchestrated nondisclosure agreements. And to make matters worse, at Biogen my old roommate and friend Bill Rastetter had recently retired as CEO.

I'd later learn that negotiations between Genentech and Biogen had reached a stalemate, and there was no clear path forward. King Kong versus Rodan. I imagined a battle taking place behind the scenes, in closed boardrooms, with pinstriped lawyers. At stake was who would be on the hook for an $800 million clinical trial of B cell therapy for MS and how would a $40 billion annual market for MS drugs be carved up and protected? The scientists who made the basic discoveries, the government agencies and private foundations that paid for essential lab work, and the patients whose lives were held in the balance were nowhere in sight.

I had to assume that Biogen's first priority was to protect the franchise. Why compete with yourself? However, there were also other, very reasonable concerns about the viability of rituximab for MS. There was simply not enough time left on the clock for the drug to turn enough profit to recoup the huge costs required for large-scale clinical trials in MS. Drugs only have a 21-year patent, even when put to new uses, and rituximab's was set to expire in 2013. It was possible to extend the patent for five years in the United States only, but even then, the calculus was unfavorable. Also, since the drug had been in use against cancer for a decade, it was far too cheap by current standards, and there was no easy way to raise the price dramatically without incurring the wrath of patients and insurers. And generic competitors, like vultures circling the old lion, were already rolling out copycats, cheaper versions of rituximab ready to hit the market the moment the patent expired. Bottom line, new clinical trials in MS made little commercial sense for either company. Knowing all this, Genentech's decision to fund the earlier rituximab trial was even more inspiring to me; they were truly acting in the public's interest.

There was more. In the original co-development agreement between IDEC and Genentech, the language stipulated that if Genentech made their own new B cell–targeted drug, the deal changed. IDEC would then receive a lower percentage of the profits, not just for the new drug but also for rituximab. Biogen's losses would be estimated, conservatively, at a billion dollars a year. It would be great for Genentech but terrible for Biogen. So Genentech went ahead and did exactly that.

Genentech's new B cell–targeted drug, named ocrelizumab, was reengineered to be even better than rituximab. A mouthful to say but, at least in theory, far more attractive—ocrelizumab was modern in design with even less mouse protein and with other more favorable characteristics.*

And if all of this wasn't enough, Roche then bought Genentech.† Swallowed it whole. Prior to the purchase, Roche had already been the majority—but pretty much hands-off—owner of Genentech. However, Roche would now fully integrate Genentech into its organization. Genentech was an iconic Northern California behemoth that still thought of itself as an irreverent, disruptive start-up. Risk-takers, proud of their reputation as Silicon Valley cowboys, they aimed to make a difference in people's lives no matter the cost.‡ Genentech was aggressive; their mantra was to make decisions rapidly and move forward. Roche was the opposite: a conservative, family-owned Swiss firm built on consensus. The cultures of the two companies could not have been more different.

Still, Roche had also been in the rituximab business nearly from the beginning. It was Roche that first brought to IDEC the idea of testing a B cell therapy for rheumatoid arthritis. They funded the original rituximab trial for arthritis and had global development rights for all non-cancer indications, now including MS. But there were too many reasons why rituximab would never be formally developed for MS. As an early biotech product, it was too cheap to justify the cost of large clinical trials, its patent life would soon expire, and even cheaper generics were on the way.

---

* Ocrelizumab kills B cells mostly using other cells (a mechanism known as antibody-dependent cell-mediated cytotoxicity, or ADCC) rather than complement proteins, which is likely to lessen side effects in patients compared to rituximab.

† Roche had purchased a majority stake in Genentech in 1990; the outright acquisition occurred in 2009.

‡ The full story, as with all myths, is somewhat more nuanced, as it includes allegations that Genentech's first product was based on a DNA sample taken from a UCSF lab in the middle of the night (Dalton, R., Schiermeier, Q. "Genentech pays $200m over growth hormone 'theft'." *Nature* 402, 335, 1999).

And worse yet, even if Genentech's new drug worked, insurers, patients, and physicians alike might simply opt for the older drug rituximab that could be purchased for a tenth of the cost. Why buy a Rolls when a Volkswagen works nearly as well?

None of this was transparent to the academic partners or evident to the patients. I was narrowly focused on completing the trials, obtaining FDA approval, getting a revolutionary therapy to as many people as possible as quickly as possible, and understanding the biology of how it worked. I was living in an ivory tower.

* * *

Just as my frustration neared a boiling point, the logjam suddenly eased. The ink was barely dry on Roche's acquisition of Genentech when I received a call from the new director of neuroscience at Roche.

"Steve, I have great news. Our board of directors has approved funding for an MS study with ocrelizumab. We'd like to meet as soon as possible, with you and Ludwig Kappos, to discuss the details."

Hallelujah. I nearly fell off my chair.

Kappos was Europe's most seasoned expert in MS clinical trials. Based in Basel, just down the road from Roche, he had a long history of working with the company, just as I had with Genentech in Northern California. We liked and respected each other. More important, Ludwig's knowledge of the landscape of MS therapeutics was unrivaled, and I knew that he was unafraid to express his views forcefully and argue for the best possible studies. He proved to be the ideal partner for everything that followed.

Roche had moved suddenly and in a most impressive fashion. They quietly came to an agreement with Biogen, behind the scenes and out of the press, wresting control of the commercial anti-CD20 B cell franchise. And our MS program was again on the launchpad. I'd never have guessed that this giant pharmaceutical company, known for its Swiss caution, would have been able to act so quickly or decisively.

This momentous decision was not driven by financial calculations alone. I knew that Roche believed that they had an ethical obligation to move forward. Genentech, their former partner and now subsidiary, was certainly campaigning on behalf of our program, but now the ultimate decision-making authority rested in Basel and not South San Francisco. The leaders at Roche independently concluded that the rituximab MS data were so profound that they had to follow up with some therapy of this type, despite the uncertain financial payoff for the company. I believed that two programs should be advanced together, one with the known drug rituximab that could reach patients within a few years, and a second with ocrelizumab, a longer play that first needed preliminary testing. In this way, patients would benefit as quickly as possible from rituximab, and if the new drug was as good as we hoped, it could take over down the road. I argued strongly for this two-drug strategy.

But then the FDA stepped in—again. They ordered us to test different doses of rituximab before beginning any final study. More than two million doses of rituximab had been given since it was first approved to treat blood cancer. We already knew the dose needed to kill B cells in the bloodstream, and even though our MS study was modest in size, the results were clear and convincing.

We could have pushed back and fought with the bureaucrats at the FDA, but that would have consumed precious time, and we were likely to lose anyway. So bottom line was that rituximab could not be officially brought to the marketplace for MS any sooner than the new drug. Each required more preliminary testing before a final pivotal trial could be started. Faced with this reality, our choice was now clear. We'd move forward with the better version of our drug, ocrelizumab. The glass was only half full, but at least we were back in the game.

We'd begin by testing more than one dose. We were flying blind but ultimately chose two doses, one matching the rituximab dose, and the other a lower dose.

The trial was designed to replicate our earlier study with rituximab, but was more complex. Instead of two treatment groups, or arms, there would be four groups of 60 patients each—this would satisfy the need to test more than one dose. One group would receive a placebo, two others a high or low dose of the new drug administered by infusion into a vein. The surprising fourth arm was Biogen's minimally effective beta interferon drug administered by injections directly into muscle. If the new drug worked as expected, interferon as a treatment for MS would be a thing of the past.

It was also possible, however, that ocrelizumab would fail. Although the new drug attaches to the same protein on B cells as rituximab does, the similarities end there. The two drugs bind different sites on the protein, reach different areas of the body, and kill B cells mostly in different ways.

Antibodies are often compared with bullets, but bullets are packed with energy and destroy victims on their own, while antibodies and antibody drugs require outside help to accomplish the task. When an antibody attaches to a cell, the cell can be killed in one of two ways: by proteins called complement, or by special immune system troops.

Complement punches holes in the wall of the cell, which then takes on water and dies like a sinking *Titanic*. Immune system killers work by attaching to the rear of an antibody that is bound to another cell, piggyback style, then releasing substances that destroy the cell membrane. Old friend rituximab kills chiefly through complement, while ocrelizumab works mostly the other way. It was possible that the new drug might be better at killing cells outside the bloodstream, deep in hidden niches of the body, in the lymph nodes, spleen, and liver.

So even though the two drugs kill the same type of cell (the B cell) by attaching to the same protein (CD20), the way they seek out and destroy B cells in the body is very different. It would not have been at all surprising if the two drugs had radically different effects on MS.

We started the trial. For more than a year, everything went smoothly. But then it happened. A black swan.

CHAPTER 35

A Black Swan Incident

Early on a June morning in 2009, just as soon as the caffeine took hold, I began my daily ritual of scrolling through my inbox, deleting scores of messages that had somehow wiggled past the spam filters to find the few important ones. Today was no different, except that one message packed a wallop. Roche headquarters asked me to call immediately.

It had to be a problem of the very worst kind.

When I called, I learned that a patient enrolled in the MS trial had died under highly worrisome circumstances. Patient 405, a 41-year-old woman with typical relapsing MS that had begun 10 years earlier. Twelve weeks into the study, she underwent routine blood and MRI follow-up studies that were all unremarkable. Several hours after leaving the clinic, however, she developed confusion, then delirium and seizures. Her husband rushed her to the local emergency room, where her seizures were treated successfully, and by the next day she seemed to have recovered. However, later that day she rapidly deteriorated and was soon critically ill, with a high fever and dangerously low levels of platelets, which are essential for blood-clotting.* Over the next 48 hours, her brain swelled, and her liver and kidneys shut down. Despite therapy to support her bodily functions, restore platelets,

* A deficiency of platelets is known as thrombocytopenia.

suppress an overactive immune system, and treat any undiagnosed infection, her condition deteriorated to coma, cardiovascular collapse, and then death.

Unexpected deaths obviously happen not only in clinical trials but also in real life, and sometimes it's hard to pin down their cause. The difficulty with a clinical trial is that you often don't immediately know if the event is related to the drug being tested. Worse yet, when something like this happens, it could be a harbinger of more to come. So the challenge is to move as quickly as possible to determine if the study drug was responsible while protecting as best you can the many other patients receiving the experimental treatment.

The most notable example of a disastrous complication due to an MS drug occurred with natalizumab, the monoclonal antibody treatment that works by blocking movement of immune cells into the brain. Shortly after its launch, the drug was removed from the market when patients developed a horrific viral infection of the brain.* Eventually, a blood test was developed that identified people at risk for this complication, permitting the return of natalizumab to the market.†

But it was a complication from a different MS drug that resonated eerily and even more deeply. During clinical trials with alemtuzumab, a powerful immunosuppressant drug, two patients developed a severe drop in platelets, leading to uncontrolled bleeding and ultimately death. Autopsies of the victims revealed fulminant autoimmune disease. Their immune systems had attacked and destroyed the body's platelets, misinterpreting them as foreign invaders.‡

It was soon recognized that many other patients treated with

---

* Progressive multifocal leukoencephalopathy, or PML.

† With screening for PML risk, approximately half of MS patients can now be safely treated with natalizumab.

‡ A disorder known as immune thrombocytopenic purpura.

alemtuzumab also developed low but not life-threatening platelet levels, leaving little doubt that the drug was responsible. And there was more. About a quarter of the patients developed an autoimmune disease of the thyroid gland called Graves' disease. Amazingly, alemtuzumab had been used in bone marrow transplantation for many years without any hint that thyroid issues might arise. Clearly, people with MS were at special risk for this complication. They were autoimmune prone.

I was extremely concerned that something similar might have happened to patient 405. It was biologically plausible and very frightening.

Our first priority was to unblind the treatment that she received; perhaps it was placebo or interferon, in which case our drug could not be implicated. But we learned she had received ocrelizumab, and worse yet, was in the high dose group.

Patient 405's doctors had been unable to establish the cause of her illness and death. An autopsy had been done, and tissues sent to an outside pathologist in an effort to identify what happened, but even this had not produced an answer. We needed to know everything possible about this patient to understand if she died from ocrelizumab or from some unrelated cause. An unexplained death during our clinical trial could bring B cell therapy for MS to a screeching halt.

After speaking with her physician by phone, we also learned that five days earlier she'd been strolling with her husband in a downtown park and was stung by a bee on her forehead, causing progressively worsening swelling of her face. Maybe the bee sting and not our drug was responsible.

Had she arrived in an academic medical center in Boston, Baltimore, London, Paris, Berlin, Warsaw, Tokyo, or any of dozens of places around the globe, getting to the bottom of the problem would have been so much easier. We might have known the doctors personally; they'd likely have reached out to ask for our help in the first place. This patient, however, lived in Novi Sad, a small city in north-central Serbia, which made it more challenging to investigate the death.

Today the vast majority of modern clinical trials are conducted across the globe, a sea change from the situation a generation ago when patients were usually from North America and Western Europe. The ocrelizumab trials enrolled more than 2,500 patients from more than 90 nations around the world. Global trials bring many advantages, including more rapid enrollment, reduced costs, and networks of physicians and scientists who learn from each other and work in concert for the betterment of health—true global communities. But there are also potential disadvantages, especially when one needs to troubleshoot in unfamiliar medical systems.

David Leppert, who had just arrived at Roche, was now charged with oversight of the drug trials. A former postdoctoral fellow in my lab, David had extensive experience in B cell therapeutics and helped lead the original rituximab studies at Genentech. David quickly concluded, correctly, that this incident created a threat to the entire B cell therapy program, and that more should be done in an attempt to find out what had happened. He began by speaking with the local Serbian-speaking data monitor. Data monitors are the compliance officers for clinical trials. They ensure that each center obeys all requirements for human research at their institution, completes data entry, maintains full records, implements the study protocol exactly, and cares for each patient in a medically and ethically responsible manner. Data monitoring is usually provided as part of a menu of services contracted through large clinical research organizations (CROs). These corporations support the efficient conduct of clinical trials. They employ full-time specialists across the globe, including teams of data monitors, often individuals who know the clinicians they help select for the new study.

Next, Leppert's team traveled to Novi Sad to meet with the data monitor and neurologist in person and to review relevant medical data. They scrutinized the patient's medical records, obtained stored tissue samples for additional analyses, and performed further testing on blood samples, including genetic tests, to help clarify the cause of death. But no sign of any infection, preexisting medical condition, or predisposition could be found. These studies were immensely helpful to exclude many causes of sudden demise, but they also failed to pinpoint what happened to patient 405.

We advanced a working diagnosis of systemic inflammatory response syndrome (SIRS). The term "syndrome" means that this type of thing has been seen before; it implies that there could be many causes, or that the cause is entirely unknown. SIRS describes an overactive inflammatory response affecting many organs of the body. It can follow infections, vaccinations, bites (such as bee stings), cancer, or sometimes occurs without any evident cause. A diagnosis of SIRS permitted us to exclude the autoimmune platelet disorder seen with the other MS drug as the cause of death.

Here the trail ended, and we were left with uncertainty. If no additional cases appeared, we could reasonably, if tentatively, conclude that this was an isolated event. We were cautiously optimistic that the new drug was not the offender, but we could not be sure. An aphorism taught to every young scientist is that one cannot prove a negative. The only way to be reasonably confident that other patients would not experience terrible events similar to patient 405's was to treat many more—thousands more—monitor carefully, cross our fingers, and see what happened.

CHAPTER 36

Government Service

In the midst of all this, one busy Monday in 2009, after I'd made hospital rounds with the residents and students in the morning, saw my personal patients in clinic all afternoon, then ran to an early evening meeting with the other department chairs, I returned to my office just past 7:00 p.m. As usual, a half-inch stack of new messages was on my desk, plus a few hundred emails in my inbox, and a pile of snail mail letters, books, and manuscripts for review. I flipped through the phone messages. Routine issues—patient issues that couldn't be answered by the on-call residents or clinic nurses, a few scientific inquiries, a couple of salespeople. And the White House.

I assumed that the call from the White House was a request to meet with a dignitary, as occasionally happened—I'd call in the morning after first making sure it wasn't a mistake. Tuesday was as busy as Monday, though, and I spent the entire day in the hospital with the residents and a group of new patients who'd been admitted overnight. I'd completely forgotten about the White House's call until it came up at my staff meeting the following day.

"Dr. Hauser, the White House called again, asking to speak with you. Don't you think we should return their call?"

"Yipes, it slipped my mind. I've been so busy. Did you ask them what it's about?"

"I did. They said it was a personal matter."

"OK," I said. "It's now past 7:00 p.m. in Washington. Can you connect me during my commute in the morning?"

"Of course. We'll add it to the to-do list."

I'm not a great driver. My gaze wanders. I need a horse blinder for humans.* I also get lost in thought, a trait I can't indulge in because so much work must be completed during morning and evening drives. My car is a mobile office, connected with my assistants, used for dictations, returning calls, and sometimes phone meetings. Not to mention breakfast.

The next morning, I was connected with the White House. The president wanted to advance my name, along with ten others, to serve on a bioethics commission charged with advising the administration on advances in science and medicine and their implications for society. I'd need to undergo a background check and confirm there was nothing embarrassing in my past. Also, if I should be appointed, I, and my immediate family, would need to divest ourselves of all stock and other assets valued at more than $10,000 held in any individual company that could potentially have an interest in issues that the committee might address. The cardinal rule of the new administration, I was told, would be "no surprises."

No illegal nannies in our past, no worrisome entanglements with pharmaceutical companies, no income from the drugs I helped develop. I'd be clean as a whistle, that was for sure. So over the next seven months, I underwent three rounds of background checks. They dug deeply, even uncovering that a decade earlier one of our kids had trespassed on a private golf course. It was a sledding party, with trays borrowed from the high school cafeteria, punished by a half day of cleaning detail at the police station. Otherwise, they turned up nada. So in

* Believe it or not, you can purchase these—they're manufactured by Panasonic.

early 2010, I was notified that the vetting was complete and my appointment would go forward, and several months later, the names of the new commission members were announced.

The prior bioethics commission under George W. Bush had kicked up a firestorm over the issue of stem cell research, which touched on the highly charged issue of using human fetal tissue for research. A colleague of mine at UCSF, Elizabeth Blackburn, had been fired from that commission for her stance in favor of stem cell research.

A calmer advisory group was needed, and President Barack Obama had no desire to stir up any more controversy. He had enough problems on his hands already with the economy in tatters. However, the commission was not composed of shrinking violets, nor was it monotheistic. It was chaired by Amy Gutmann, a lawyer and bioethicist and president of the University of Pennsylvania. James Wagner, an engineer and president of Emory University, served as co-chair. The other nine members of the commission included scientists, academic physicians, clergy, experts in bioethics and the law, and even a public representative, Lonnie Ali, the ex-boxing champ's wife.

A few press reports noted that we'd been selected based on a litmus test. We were committed lefties, fellow travelers favoring godless science and physician-sanctioned euthanasia ("playing God"). As summarized by the Catholic News Agency, "Every one of Obama's current advisors who has written on bioethical issues 'is pro-abortion, pro-embryonic stem cell research, pro-euthanasia, pro-assisted suicide. Bioethicists like this strive to create a "Brave New World" for the weakest and most vulnerable of those created in God's image: those who doctors used to swear an oath to protect.'"*

---

* Catholic News Agency, December 5, 2009, quoting Rev. Thomas J. Euteneuer.

In fact, I was a registered Republican at the time, and later learned that several other commission members were as well.

Service on the commission was intense but enormously gratifying. We examined and published reports on many topics, including the risks and benefits of synthetic biology—creating life in a test tube—and ethical issues resulting from genome sequencing and advances in molecular biology.

We investigated a gruesome mid-20th-century US-sponsored debacle in Guatemala that had recently come to light, where vulnerable populations were inoculated with syphilis and other sexually transmitted organisms, sometimes directly into their nervous systems, without their consent. This led us to next review the adequacy of ethical standards for protection of participants in human research, nationally and globally. We weighed in on vaccine preparedness for public health emergencies, bioterrorism, and research in children.

Unfortunately, we didn't tackle the subject that commission member John Arras wisely called "the bioethical issue of our time," healthcare. During its first term, the Obama White House requested that we not address healthcare because of sensitivity surrounding the pending Affordable Care Act legislation, aka Obamacare. Our commission's charter permitted us to overrule this request, but such an act would have been self-defeating. Had we pushed ahead, we might have silenced our voice in the administration. We'd certainly have lessened our impact. So, we tabled a discussion of healthcare, planning to reanimate it after the 2012 elections. But this never happened. Other urgent tasks appeared, including some related to bioterrorism. The closest we came to tackling healthcare was a study of incidental findings in medicine.

Incidental findings are unexpected ones. These have proliferated as technologies advance to examine the body in astounding detail—to image organs, monitor functions, map genes, and measure chemistries. A patient complains of shortness of breath, and a chest MRI scan shows an unrelated cyst in a rib. Or, as part of a general checkup, hundreds of blood tests are ordered "just to be sure," and a couple are mildly outside the range of normal.

Following up on findings such as these makes healthcare more complicated, more costly, and sometimes more dangerous to patients. To illustrate the problem, we highlighted cases from real life. One involved an elderly man who underwent unnecessary surgery for a benign spot on his lung, and suffered terrible postoperative complications. In general terms, we took the position that it was OK not to look for incidental findings and argued against use of unfocused diagnostic evaluations and bundled aggregates of tests.

The commission worked in a fishbowl. Meetings were announced in advance, open to the public, and disseminated via video stream. Interested individuals and groups had forewarning and could pack the audience. Most were concerned citizens hoping to educate and influence commission members around issues related to our studies and reports. Decent, concerned citizens. For example, during our deliberations on protection for participants in clinical research, we heard from individuals who suffered life-threatening complications from experimental treatment and then learned they were held responsible for the medical bills.*

Another example of useful public participation was during our study of synthetic biology and the claim—unfounded—that life had been created in a test tube. Here, we heard diverse views from individuals concerned that this new science was immoral,

---

* This seemed outrageous to me, but there is another side of the argument. If researchers are required to indemnify research participants, we were told, the costs of clinical research would skyrocket, and the pace of medical progress would slow. On this point, members of the commission were divided, but I remain on the side that supports the guarantee of free medical care for injuries sustained from participation in clinical research.

sacrilegious, or dangerous to global ecosystems. These comments broadened our perspective considerably.

The president planned to launch an ambitious multibillion-dollar neuroscience initiative and asked our commission to weigh in and advise.* Organized groups concerned about government surveillance descended on us. The largest, an outfit named Freedom from Covert Harassment and Surveillance, was led by an attorney who looked, dressed, and otherwise seemed quite normal, except of course that he seemed to buy into the whole obsession. This guy believed that selected individuals were being targeted for brainwashing and mind control by the US government. He functioned as the magnet connecting petitioners around the country and bringing them together into our midst. It reached a crescendo at a commission meeting at the Warwick Hotel in New York City.

By federal mandate, any member of the public who wished to speak to the commission was provided 90 seconds of open mic time at the end of each meeting. Longer statements could be provided as written documents to commission staff. Here is a small sample of the public comments that day.†

> "I've been a victim of ongoing nonconsensual human subject experimentation for my entire adult life, and possibly may have been a victim since my childhood. I have been targeted with ongoing microwave weapons, as well as drugging with neurotoxic contaminants covertly placed on articles of clothing, as well as on other personal possessions. I believe my being a nonconsensual human test subject is related to the CIA's MK Alter Behavior Modification Program that . . . emphasized that it would be necessary to test un-

* The US Brain Research Through Advancing Innovative Neurotechnologies (BRAIN) Initiative.

† The Presidential Commission for the Study of Bioethical Issues, https://bioethicsarchive.georgetown.edu/pcsbi/node/225.html.

> witting citizens in their ordinary day activities without their knowledge in the final stage of the testing program. . . . [O]ther members of my family . . . were victims also."
>
> "I have been and continue to be experimented on against my will and without my permission as a human test subject and as a targeted individual forced into trauma-based mind control programs. . . . My left arm occasionally experiences pain and discomfort from an object of unknown origin moving under my skin and being activated somehow. I have an unusual dental filling of unknown origin on the side of one of my back upper right teeth and no memory of having this procedure done."

Others described similar experiences and fears. How could we even begin to deal with this? On the surface, these people seemed more or less normal. Anxious certainly, but not particularly disheveled or confused. No overt hallucinations. Their paranoia seemed mostly an isolated symptom, something medically classified as a cluster A personality disorder. Individually, they seemed almost reasonable, but when grouped together, their fears were reinforced, and anxiety bubbled up into aggression.

We needed protection and were quickly assigned a security detail. Special entrances and exits were developed for us, and metal detectors were installed to screen attendees at the meeting rooms. The most disconcerting moment was when two large men in suits rose in unison, walked in front of the table where we were sitting, and demanded that we cease electronic harassment. One suddenly reached into his chest pocket and began to pull something out. Certain that it was a gun, we ducked. The security detail jumped forward. The cameras were rolling—all of our meetings were broadcast. I had visions of a public assassination played out on the evening news. But instead of a weapon, he brandished only a written manifesto to read to us.

The activities of these groups soon spread beyond the meeting venues. One commission member received a threatening package anonymously placed at the front door of his home. He'd been assured that his home address was securely protected from discovery. The package was found by his two young children. Thankfully, the bomb squad found that the package was empty. It was a false alarm, but one with clear malevolent intent. A warning, perhaps, and if the goal was to frighten commission members, the unknown perpetrators were successful.

A California-based contingent went after me.

"Hauser, stop supporting electronic surveillance," they'd shout in the hospital lobby.

On one occasion, several arrived at my office in a state of agitation, demanding that I stop the government from brainwashing their kids. Police were summoned, and they were led away peacefully. Fortunately, over time, as the commission moved on to other topics, these groups also moved on, focusing their attention on others who might advance their goals more effectively than we could.

A postscript: At the end of the Obama presidency, most commission members resigned voluntarily. By tradition, each new president selects his or her own bioethics commission, always with new members, so this action made sense. But I decided not to resign, along with one other commission member. Perhaps the new president would wish to have our counsel. He might need help with ethics even more than his predecessors did.

But Donald J. Trump decided he did not need bioethics advice in any form whatsoever. And after two years of silence, we received a note from the White House informing us that our services were no longer needed.

CHAPTER 37

Another Close Call

We completed the phase 2 preliminary study of ocrelizumab in early December 2009. More than three years had passed since the end of the rituximab trial, three years on a roller coaster, waves of exhilaration and deep disappointments. But finally, somehow, we'd made it to the next level. And when we saw the results, there for the first time, we were thrilled. Thrilled and flabbergasted. All of the delays, anxieties, and uncertainties were now in the rearview mirror.

The results were jaw-dropping—a near-complete absence of new brain inflammation in patients with relapsing MS who received ocrelizumab, but not in those treated with placebo or Biogen's interferon drug. To top that off, the low dose of the drug performed as well as the high dose. And no new serious safety concerns emerged. A trifecta. Ocrelizumab was easily as effective as rituximab.

There was even more good news. When the drug was out of the patient's system, there was no sign of "rebound," a dangerous flare-up of brain inflammation that can occur when some other MS drugs are discontinued.* And even long after B cells

* "Rebound" can occur after stopping MS therapies that block movement of immune cells from the bloodstream to brain. Natalizumab (Tysabri) and dimethyl fumarate (Gilenya) are MS drugs in this category. With these drugs, large numbers of autoimmune cells are stuck in place at the entrance of the brain, and when the drug is

had returned to the bloodstream, MS remained in complete remission.

Silent. Like Elvis, MS had left the building. We saw hints of this in the earlier rituximab study, but now here it was, no question, in 3D Technicolor. Not only was MS suppressed, but maybe the immune system was rebooted as well. If it was, then short-term treatment might confer long-term protection.

This last bit of news made me especially happy, but it was, in truth, possibly a problem for our pharmaceutical partners. Short-term treatment would mean less drug sold. I was concerned that a lower projection of ocrelizumab's commercial potential could tip the scales against moving forward.

Nonetheless, these new data, combined with the earlier rituximab results, were simply too powerful to not proceed with phase 3 trials. However, it was still uncertain how these would proceed. The phase 2 trial inflamed an already contentious relationship between Biogen and Roche/Genentech. I believed that Biogen's strategy was to continue to delay any decision regarding the new drug and push instead for development of the old drug, rituximab, a compound with a royalty split more favorable to them.

A summit took place in early 2010 at Biogen headquarters in Cambridge, Massachusetts, attended by representatives of Roche and Genentech, now a single, but still not yet completely harmonious, entity. It was a closed meeting that excluded the academic partners, including me. The purpose was to see what a final, phase 3 MS study would look like. Biogen's position, unchanged from before the first ocrelizumab trial, was not unreasonable. Why bother to go with ocrelizumab when rituximab is around?

---

stopped, the gates open, and violent inflammation can occur. We were confident that rebound would not occur with ocrelizumab because it killed the culprit cells. The bad actors were not on the tarmac; they were destroyed. But we needed real data to be sure, and now we had the proof.

We know so much more about rituximab; after all, two million people have been treated over more than two decades. Furthermore, the long-term safety of the new drug was still uncertain—remember patient 405. And the final arrow in Biogen's quiver was that the new drug would never be commercially viable unless it was priced similar to rituximab, which was already inexpensive and, due to its expiring patent, would soon be faced with competition from even cheaper generic copycats.

If the new drug worked better, this could justify a higher price, but the earlier rituximab results were so overwhelmingly positive that the bar was already set at an impossibly high level. Perhaps one could charge whatever price one wished, but there was always the risk that MS patients—and their physicians and insurers—would choose rituximab over a far more expensive new version.

Roche, though, was secure in the driver's seat. They'd go forward with ocrelizumab. Rituximab was old news. The new drug was just too promising to pass on. It was a more modern drug that would be safer with repeated use. The preliminary studies suggested that it worked as well and maybe even better than rituximab, and it made commercial sense. It could add billions of dollars annually to Roche's bottom line. And only ocrelizumab had been tested at different doses as the FDA had demanded, so pivotal phase 3 studies could move forward immediately. The lower dose was chosen for the final trials. I had argued for this choice, believing that the preliminary trials showed no meaningful differences between the two doses that were tested, and was thus delighted with this decision.

But, once again, my joy was to be short-lived.

* * *

The next tsunami struck at the worst possible moment, in February 2010. Something had gone terribly wrong in a different study of ocrelizumab. A safety problem in patients with rheumatoid arthritis. Rituximab was known to work modestly well in rheumatoid arthritis, though not nearly as well as in MS. The scientists at Roche thought that maybe ocrelizumab would work better, especially if they increased the dose. So they tried it. I wish they hadn't.

Thirteen cases of unusual infections occurred, all in patients from Southeast Asia treated with the high dose of the new drug. There was no specific pattern, and most were common infections that normally occur in this region of Asia, except of course they were happening at a higher-than-expected frequency. Tuberculosis, fungus, other rare bugs. An analysis suggested that, in addition to the high dose, old age, longstanding use of immune suppressants, and other coexisting illnesses may have been responsible. Thirteen cases, from a study that had nothing to do with MS, in patients who in no way resembled people with MS. But maybe this would be enough to doom the most promising approach ever developed for MS.

The news came just as we were setting in motion the final push forward for the MS program. The merger between Roche and Genentech was still very much a work in progress. A decision was quickly made that all further studies of ocrelizumab in rheumatoid arthritis were to be canceled immediately, a decree that came from central command at Roche.

The scientists at Genentech were crestfallen. How could this have happened? In their view, pulling the plug on the arthritis trial was not based on in-depth analysis of data. Why were they not consulted? The decision was wildly premature, they argued. The complete data was not even available when the program was halted.

Economic considerations might have played a role in the decision. Ocrelizumab would be expensive. The arthritis community—patients, clinicians, and insurers—had grown accustomed to paying low prices for rituximab, and they were unlikely to pay much more for a shiny new model. Everyone knew that B cell therapy offered only modest benefits in rheumatoid arthritis; it was used as an add-on to other drugs, not as first-line treatment. The benefits for arthritis were nothing like the spectacular results seen in MS.

MS drugs were already notoriously expensive. Sky-high drug prices were the norm. So better to keep the two drugs separate: stick with cheap rituximab for arthritis, and develop the costly new drug only for MS. This would be less confusing, and the value of the MS franchise would be protected.

The patients with infections all recovered uneventfully, and no new cases appeared. Thank goodness. A few more black hairs turned gray, but the most important thing was that we'd safely traversed another bump in the road. At long last, we had a green light to complete the phase 3 testing of ocrelizumab, two identical trials in relapsing MS and a third in the primary progressive form of the disease.

An $800 million experiment to prove beyond doubt that B cell therapy unequivocally worked against MS.

CHAPTER 38

The Problem of Progression

We are born with 100 billion nerve cells in our brain, more or less. But beginning in our early twenties, we lose about a million each day. And they don't grow back. It's a sad fact of life. Fortunately, we really don't need, or use, all of them.

Women have smaller brains than men, and fewer numbers of cortical neurons—brain cells near the surface that do the really important things like thinking—but this is not necessarily a disadvantage. Size doesn't matter. Elephants have huge brains, much larger than those of humans, but there are no elephants at Harvard, except for a few skeletons at the Agassiz Museum. What does matter is how effectively brain cells are used, and especially how well they connect with other cells, near and far. The ratio of brain weight to total body mass roughly correlates with intelligence, and here the average woman is better endowed than her typical male colleague. She has more brain per pound.

No matter where one's brain begins, however, a daily loss of nerve cells sooner or later will take its toll over time, even though the age at which this becomes noticeable depends on what we ask our brains to do. Power hitters in baseball have difficulty turning on fastballs when they reach their mid-thirties. In tennis, the fall-off is even earlier, usually by the mid-twenties. For weekend warriors, age-related declines don't become apparent until much later, unless you are going against your college-age kids in *Jeopardy!* or testing your hand-eye coordination against theirs on a video game. Still, in many academic, business, or social circles, elders often win due to combinations of experience, judgment, attention to detail, and, maybe, cunning.

People with MS are also losing brain cells like the rest of us, but at a much faster rate: three million cells per day. When a person loses 1 percent or so of brain cells every year, sooner or later it becomes noticeable. Brain fog, fatigue, imbalance, and urinary urgency are near-universal complaints in people with MS, even in people who are otherwise doing well. But sometimes, even without treatment of any kind, MS causes little or no disability at all.

* * *

I was asked to see Helen, an 85-year-old woman who'd been suffering from headaches throughout her adult life. Her internist of many years had retired, and the new physician decided to obtain an MRI scan "just to make sure that everything was OK." Well, the MRI showed that she had MS. And not a little bit of MS, lots of it, scars throughout her brain.

I love seeing older people, especially the spirited ones, like Helen. After a few minutes together, it became clear that her headaches were due to migraine, nothing more. I could prescribe a treatment to prevent attacks, in a very low dose given her age, and she'd be fine. Case closed. But what about the MRI? Had she ever experienced other neurologic symptoms?

"Oh, yes, young man,"* she replied. "Often. I have multiple sclerosis, you see. It started with blurred vision when I was in college. I've had times with numbness, a little imbalance;

---

* I was in my sixties at the time.

sometimes I feel very tired. My bladder doesn't work well, but many women my age have this problem. Most of my friends complain about the same thing. It might be due to my pregnancies or maybe it's my MS. I'm really not sure. Anyway, I just live with it, and when my body starts growling at me, I just bark back. It's really no big thing."

Is it possible for people to have just a touch of MS, just as others have a touch of arthritis? Yes, indeed. Sometimes MS is so mild that it never announces itself at all. It just lies dormant, causing no trouble.

When I meet people like Helen—and I've met scores of them—people who've had MS for many decades, received little or no treatment, and are without any disability, they often have one thing in common. They're tough. They have an arrogance toward the disease, more important things to do, no time to deal with the nuisance. They never give in. But when MS hits hard, as it more often does, a positive mindset alone is not nearly enough. MS is a cruel master that can checkmate the strongest will to win.

* * *

Charlie was my friend and patient. He was a brilliant, charismatic, top-drawer surgical resident at Harvard. He also had terrible MS. It began, tragically, as it so often does, at liftoff, just as his career was beginning. And he fought it like the dickens. Never missed an on-call night, no matter how tired or ill he was. Until a loss of coordination no longer made it safe to practice surgery. So, he became an educator and was soon voted best teacher in the entire medical school. He'd hold rounds at 6:00 a.m. The students knew that it was well worth setting their alarm clocks early to be there. He made it in every day, even though it took hours to get ready for work, and whenever someone asked Charlie how he was feeling, he'd answer, "It's a beautiful day!"

His wife and daughter adored him, as did everyone else. Charlie continued for as long as he possibly could, until the march of the disease took its toll. Near the end, nothing worked any longer; no part of his body would obey the brain's commands. He died far too young at age 60. Charlie was the most optimistic, good-natured human being one could ever meet. But the MS won. So inner strength will only take you so far. If you are on the fence, it might swing you to the side of health. But when MS digs in hard, the body will lose the fight, no matter how much optimism the host can muster.

* * *

Why is MS mild in some people and devastating in others? Bursts of inflammation in the MS brain vary from patient to patient. They are sometimes placid, often angry, occasionally catastrophic. Each is unique. Many are in "silent" areas of the brain, areas not being used, at least not consciously so, but over time these disrupt the thousand or so major cable wire systems that encode our experiences and regulate the behaviors, emotions, and desires that make us who we are. With each MS attack, the brain loses some of its reserve and becomes less flexible as it responds to injury. The battery drains.

Also important is the body's resilience: its resistance to injury and capacity for self-repair. The damage to myelin in MS is often followed by repair—like a tadpole that regrows its severed tail. But repaired myelin is never as good as the original. It is skinny and fragile; it short-circuits and burns out under stress or heavy work demands. A permanent rent in the fabric of the brain.

A recipe for a hardy brain is a healthy lifestyle, no earlier injuries, and, especially, favorable genetics—choose your parents wisely. And if you want to get better, it is always best to be young. You'll have less damage and better repair. So, plan to have your next brain attack before you get too old.

* * *

The worst problem in MS, and every patient's greatest fear, is that progressive MS will take hold. Inner strength, youth, and good health aren't enough to protect a patient from progression. This is different from the more typical relapsing MS, where patients have sudden attacks of worsening, often followed by significant recovery. By contrast, patients with progressive MS notice, gradually at first, that they are becoming steadily weaker, inexorably, week after week, year after year, a slow burn with no let-up, from limp to cane to walker to wheelchair until bedbound, socially isolated, life irreparably smashed. Without treatment, about half of patients with relapsing MS evolve into progressive MS within 15 years of onset, and less commonly symptoms are progressive from onset, the form known as Primary Progressive MS.*

Progressive MS is a guillotine hanging over the head.

* * *

When patients with MS were first treated with rituximab, the first-generation B cell therapy drug, and we saw a near-complete shutdown of brain inflammation, I had hopes that the dragon of progressive MS had been slain, at least for those who hadn't yet developed progression. And indeed, this seemed to be true for many. They continued to do well, with no new symptoms, for many years. They remained in remission and, equally import-

---

* Approximately 10% of patients with MS have the Primary Progressive form of the disease.

ant, they felt well. Some were even better than before treatment began; their brains were healing.

But not everyone.

A few rituximab-treated patients with relapsing MS began to report that they were worsening, not with sudden attacks but gradually, incrementally, inexorably. Insidious progression in people we thought had been cured. They lose balance with quick turns during a soccer match, can no longer sew because a hand becomes shaky. With fatigue, they have double vision; or while sleeping, the urine begins to leak just a little bit.

But the MRI scans show no changes. The scars in the myelin, the *sine qua non* for MS, are unchanged. No new brain lesions have formed, and shrinkage of the brain is no longer accelerating.

"How can I be getting worse," they ask, "since my MRI looks the same?"

The attacks that we thought were the sole cause of MS turn out to be the cannon fire, loud and booming, inflicting great damage, but not the whole story. When the cannons are silenced, with rituximab for example, the infantry is still there, camouflaged, lying low, hidden in brush and behind trees, but advancing silently towards their target. Small clusters of infiltrating B cells have taken up residence in the tissue lining just outside the surface of the brain, and in the spaces around penetrating blood vessels. Hiding in foxholes, underneath the skull, in small groups, protected from our missiles, from our drugs, and wounding the nerve cells underneath. Guerrilla-style. Invisible, even to our most advanced MRI scanners. We did not even know that they existed.

We don't know exactly what bullets are being fired, but prime suspects are immune chemicals or antibodies, our old friend, manufactured by B cells. They are also fomenting discontent with neighbors, educating other immune cells, T cells, and a scavenger cell called microglia to also turn against brain tissue.

Since much of this is taking place near the surface of the brain, just below the skull, the damage is nearly impossible to see on MRI scans. This explains why people with progressive MS keep getting worse even though their scans don't change much or at all. One thing that we thought we knew for sure about MS was that the inflammation was only happening in the brain and that loss of myelin was the only consequence. But now we realize that when MS becomes longstanding, the culprit B cells have now infiltrated the tissues just outside the brain, zapping our nerve cells from close range and turning on other damage-producing cells.

We were like the exterminator who sprays each room of the house with a pesticide, killing all the bugs living inside. But the spiders who live on the roof are alive and well, building nests and biting us in our sleep.

* * *

How was this missed for more than a century? The story is worth telling as a cautionary note. When the brain is examined at autopsy, we typically strip off the meninges, the tough layer of wrapping that covers the surface of the brain. It's thrown away, considered uninteresting, irrelevant. However, from time to time, fragments of the meninges are retained, stuck to the underlying brain tissue.

Way back in the 1970s, I noticed inflammation in the meningeal remnants of those long-ago MS samples and pointed this out to my mentors, expert pathologists all.

"What does this mean?" I asked.

Their answer was "postmortem artifact," meaning that lymphocytes had leaked out of the bloodstream and into the meninges only after the death of the patient.

"The inflammation has nothing to do with MS," they said. "It's seen in every brain regardless of the cause of death."

I wish I'd stuck to my guns, but I was limited by the state of science at the time and my respect for the wisdom of experts.

If we question everything, we'd have to start from scratch rather than stand on the shoulders of those who came before us. On the other hand, scientists who make the giant discoveries are often able to step back at the right moment and challenge conventional wisdom.

CHAPTER 39

Journey's End

This was a special morning. A Zoom meeting was scheduled with colleagues at Roche and Genentech to see, for the first time, results of our final ocrelizumab phase 3 trials in relapsing MS.* A press release would follow later in the day.

It was June 2015, nine years since the rituximab results first rocked the MS universe. I knew that B cell therapy worked amazingly well. Rituximab was now in use around the world for treating MS, and a growing list of scientific reports confirmed our original findings. Some of my patients had been on rituximab for more than a dozen years. And since the preliminary study with ocrelizumab was a home run, I was confident that it would work at least as well in the larger final trials. My main concern was that some new, unexpected side effect or toxicity would appear out of the blue. But the longer the trials went on, even that concern faded. I was hoping for a victory lap.

On the call were the key individuals from the company with whom I'd worked so closely these past years, the heads of neuroscience and the MS program, and the lead biostatistician who was now ready to walk us all through the results.

"Steve," he said, "as you know, we've spent the last six weeks

* The phase 3 trial of ocrelizumab in Primary Progressive MS trial was a few weeks behind, and results would have to wait until the fall.

cleaning the data, mostly entering missing information and correcting entry errors and inconsistencies. We data-locked late last week and unblinded the study, and the computers have been working all weekend. I'll share my screen. Here are the topline results completed just a few minutes ago."

I scanned a series of tables and figures crunched out by computers using the algorithms developed by our data sciences team. There were two identical studies in relapsing MS, so one could serve as a check on the other. For each result—effect on relapses, disability, MRI—the findings from the two studies were identical, confirming the validity of the results.

The tables and figures clearly revealed that the benefits of ocrelizumab were extraordinary. The new drug was not only incredibly effective but also well tolerated and—thank goodness—safe. The results were rock-solid. Ocrelizumab was a stunning success.

And a few weeks later we'd review the results of the third trial, this one in patients with Primary Progressive MS, the unusual and especially severe form that is progressive without relapses. When that study was unblinded, we saw that even patients with progressive MS benefitted: a highly significant slowing of progression was evident in those patients.* This was especially welcome news, because many drugs had been tried against this type of MS, and all had failed. Until now, with ocrelizumab.

* * *

Still, statistics don't tell the whole story. They tell us if we can be certain the results are real, that if we repeated the study 20 times, we'd find again and again that the new drug works better than the competitor. But statistics don't reveal the impact

---

* Our best estimate is that treatment produces, on average, more than seven years of continued ambulation in patients with Primary Progressive MS.

of the results; they don't tell us how meaningful the increased benefit is, if it's worth the risk, and what it's likely to mean for someone's life going forward. And they don't tell us enough about those patients, very few in number, whose MRI scans and symptoms suggested that they didn't benefit from ocrelizumab. The most important stuff lives behind the numbers. I wondered if we could look more closely into patients' individual benefits.

Way back in the 1970s, before computers, big data, MRIs, or treatments for MS, when I first tested if a chemotherapy drug that suppressed the immune system could help people with MS, the entire study consisted of 58 patients selected from two Boston hospitals, Massachusetts General and Peter Bent Brigham. I knew every patient, every detail, like the back of my hand.

But these new studies were a whole different ballgame. Nearly 2,500 patients, more than 300 hospitals on five continents, and an endless stream of data: MRIs, clinical scores, blood and spinal fluid tests, endless compliance and quality control checks—pulled together, nine million pages of information. Nobody could really get their arms around all this. It was impossible. We were in the hands of the number crunchers, the software programmers. But I still needed to find a way through the fog. I wanted to understand, in a visceral way, the experiences of patients treated with ocrelizumab. I was especially interested in learning details about the patients who didn't appear to benefit. And maybe other insights, not evident in the crunched data, would appear.

This was the art, not the science, of medicine. As scientists, we can only pay attention to the pre-specified primary goals of the clinical trial—to do otherwise causes far more harm than good. But perhaps embedded in the study were lessons from patients who had unusual responses and who might provide insights that otherwise would be lost when bundled together with 2,500 others. Such revelations might suggest how to fine-tune the drug in clinical practice or teach us something new and unexpected about MS that could be further explored in later studies.

A nagging concern was that although the rate of clinical attacks from MS plummeted with ocrelizumab, the decline was not as complete as would have been suggested from the MRI data. The brain MRI indicated that there was a new area of inflammation leading to a permanent scar in only 1 percent of patients each year, but nearly 15 percent experienced a new MS attack. How could this be possible, since we believe that attacks are caused by new areas of inflammation?* Why couldn't we see these on the MRI?

Maybe they were in the spinal cord, a region not imaged in our studies. Perhaps they were too small to be seen by MRI. Or maybe the attacks were not attacks at all. People with MS can transiently worsen when the body is stressed—by fever, infection, fatigue, hunger, or sometimes for no apparent reason at all. These "pseudo attacks" have been recognized for decades. They result from the short-circuiting of nerve impulses traveling through old scars, interrupting the transmission of signals from one part of the nervous system to another. Maybe the relapses in people taking the new drug were not real relapses at all. Perhaps they were just false alarms.

I recommended that the ocrelizumab team get together over a long weekend for a deep dive, one by one, into the medical stories of the participants who developed new symptoms or whose MRI worsened. In preparation for the meeting, we first charted, in simple figures, the course of MS in these patients throughout the duration of the trials. We displayed these, four per page, on double-sided 8.5-by-11-inch sheets,

* As noted earlier, this is unlike the situation in progressive MS, where worsening often has no MRI accompaniment.

housed in old-fashioned notebooks so that we could easily flip through the results, page by page, patient by patient. We also grouped patients by other features of interest, looking for patterns beneath the data. An inadequate approach given the large volume of data, but at least we could begin to digest the results, individually, event by event, and time interval by time interval.

It seemed fitting that the circle should be closed in New Orleans, a town so rich in memories for me. We met just off Canal Street, near the old Roosevelt Hotel, where in an earlier century my mom had interviewed John Garfield for her high school newspaper, and where a few years later she married Dad.

Beignets and coffee, pleasantries concluded, it was time to start. I opened with the most pressing question on my mind.

"Let's begin by pulling out the non-responders."

Translation: Let's look individually at the subjects who had evidence of new brain inflammation on MRI scans, or who experienced clinical attacks after receiving ocrelizumab.

Only a very small number had MRI changes, and we found that these often occurred without any associated symptoms, such as MS attacks or exceptional fatigue. Very encouraging. And when we turned our focus to symptoms, and considered each patient who clinically worsened, again we were looking at only a small number of individuals. Most attacks were minor, and many occurred within the first weeks of starting the drug, before it had reached its full effect. These attacks did not seem to reflect spinal cord involvement any more than would be expected. No red flags here either.

We then looked at disability, at the true impact of our treatment. Here we considered the entire group of study subjects. The patients who received ocrelizumab were more likely to report a better quality of life.* This was wonderful. Not only was the treatment working in our eyes, it was working in theirs also. And we also found something else that was really quite amazing; although most patients were stabilized with ocrelizumab, others actually improved on our neurologic exams—in fact, patients were 2½ times more likely to improve than worsen, and the number who improved kept increasing over time. After shutting down inflammation, the brain could begin to heal, and continue to heal over time, even when MS had been ravaging for many years. Later, additional MRI studies would show that smoldering brain degeneration, a hallmark of progressive MS and disability, also greatly improved with treatment.†

And the final flourish was an unexpected insight into the effects of the drug on MS progression. Patients with lower body weight have higher levels of the drug in their bodies, and we saw that they experienced less progression than heavier patients, without any loss of safety. Wow—this meant that higher doses of ocrelizumab might be even more effective.

These findings were even more remarkable than the first wave of results had suggested. Now we had some new questions to answer, questions that would require far longer periods of careful observation. Would the late degenerative phase of MS—progressive MS—never even develop at all? How long-lasting were the benefits? Did we need to use ocrelizumab continuously to maintain the protection? Would the drug continue to be safe over long periods of time?

My colleagues and I lobbied to continue treatment and monitoring in all patients who completed the study. We wanted

* Each subject was unaware of which treatment he or she received when the surveys were obtained.

† These innovative MRI studies were led by Douglas Arnold and his team at the Montreal Neurological Institute.

to follow every willing participant for as long as possible. This would be costly, but Roche/Genentech agreed enthusiastically with the plan and made an initial commitment for a ten-year extension study. They were living up to their motto, "doing now what patients need next."

CHAPTER 40

The Unveiling

Four months after Roche/Genentech shared the trial results on the Zoom call, the details of what we'd learned were shared with the world. It was October 9, 2015. We were in Barcelona, Spain, at the world's largest MS conference.* The huge amphitheater was filled with an audience of 6,000 people. When the doors opened, the crowd rushed forward to get the best seats, blocking the entrances. In an overflow room, 3,000 more waited expectantly, and outside, many others listened near loudspeakers placed in the hallways and courtyard of the conference center.

A front row center seat had been reserved for me, and following the introduction, I rose to the podium. I had just 12 minutes, but knew exactly what I wanted to say, and it didn't matter at all that under the harsh lights I could barely see my slides or prepared talking points. The results, projected on giant screens behind me, would speak for themselves. Cameras flashed from all corners of the room.

"Thank you, Mr. Chairman," I began. "I'm delighted to present the results of our clinical studies of a new therapy for multiple sclerosis, called ocrelizumab."

---

* The 31st Congress of the European Committee for Treatment and Research in Multiple Sclerosis (ECTRIMS).

I thanked the many people whose belief in our program had led us to that moment and then moved on to explain the biological underpinnings of the work, how we came to identify one particular cell in the immune system—the B cell—as a culprit in MS, and how we developed and tested a new class of drugs that kill B cells as an approach to treatment of all forms of the disease.

Then I displayed the spectacular results. New areas of inflammation and scarring in the brain, the hallmark of MS, were reduced by an astonishing 99 percent. Treated patients felt better, *much* better. They had less brain shrinkage, little new disability, and some even improved. And the safety data was stellar.

There was momentary silence, then sustained thunderous applause. A skeptical group, neurologists are not known for exuberant displays. Looking out from the podium, I knew that we'd hit it out of the park. So many of my friends and colleagues had worked for so many years to make this day possible, and here were results that could change the lives of millions of people worldwide. It was an extraordinary moment.

A question-and-answer session followed.

"I don't believe that you mentioned the duration of MS in the patients studied. Could you give us this information?"

"The mean duration of disease at entry into the study was approximately six and a half years and was balanced across all arms," I answered. "I displayed this on the baseline characteristics slide, which is also available online. The slide was shown only briefly, but I had twenty-three slides to cover, and you may have missed it because I needed to speak quickly. Many in the audience know that I usually speak slowly, a carryover from childhood time in Louisiana."

Laughter; the room lightened.

"Dr. Hauser, aren't you surprised that more than seventy

percent of the patients with active MS in these studies were previously untreated with any MS drug?"

"Indeed, I was surprised," I said. "But after hearing Dr. [Gavin] Giovannoni's presentation earlier today, perhaps we should not be surprised. He reported that most MS patients across the globe are not being treated with any MS drug. There are likely several reasons for this, including limited efficacy, unpleasant side effects, serious risks for some drugs, and high cost. I believe that B cell therapy could change this situation, particularly if longer follow-up of treated patients continues to show sustained benefit and safety."

As I responded to the queries, my mind kept returning to the remarkable 40-year journey of experiments and discovery that had brought me to this place, this podium, this breakthrough. And I thought of Andrea, and the many others I'd cared for over the years, who were stricken with this cruel disease too early to be helped.

CHAPTER 41

Rich Rewards

The treatment was not just effective, it was astoundingly, incredibly, preposterously effective. It nuked MS. New scars in the brain, the cause of attacks that produce the numbness, weakness, blindness, imbalance, and loss of bladder and bowel control that make MS so frightening, were nearly completely eliminated. How did this change people's lives? Dramatically.

Patients who lived in fear of attacks find that they no longer need to fret. At first, they're still not sure, still scared of the future, but over time, gradually, they have confidence that they are on the right track. No new symptoms appear and soon, on good days, they even begin to forget about the problem. It's almost as if they don't have MS at all. Even after a decade or more, the benefits and safety of B cell treatment show no sign of lessening.

For many, the only time they even think about having MS are the days when the treatment is given, by vein in a nearby clinic, and this only takes a couple of hours twice a year. They don't even have to miss a class or take off a day from work. And in time it might be possible to reduce or even stop the treatment for some because the immune system has been rebooted. The cells in the bloodstream that are allergic to myelin can no longer be detected.

And for those people who already have progressive MS, there

is finally a treatment that works, at least partially. Other MS drugs that are useful for relapsing disease were tested in people with progressive MS, and all fell short—until B cell treatment. The benefits of B-cell treatment for progressive MS are impressive, although they are still incomplete. Finding a treatment that stops progressive MS in its tracks is now the central goal of MS research.

If we can stop the autoimmune attack early enough—treat patients at the moment the disease begins, before the B cells dig in and progressive MS starts—then a cure could be in sight. And even after progression is underway, we can build a new type of missile, a more powerful one, to destroy what is left.* A new generation of therapies designed to kill or inactivate treatment-resistant B cells that hide out in the linings of the brain and cause progressive injury is being developed.

So even though progressive MS remains a challenge, especially for those with long-standing disease, we should recognize that the progress has been outstanding. Thanks to B cell therapy, relapses are securely in the rear-view mirror; people with MS can look forward to lives they never dreamed possible. Patients who were previously unable to walk without a cane or crutches 15 years after MS begins can now look forward to 40 years or longer before the ravages of MS might incapacitate. Many will never be incapacitated.

Equally exciting, we may be close to understanding what triggers B cells to injure brain tissue in the first place. The genetic studies showed that people who are predisposed to having MS inherit certain flavors of immune system genes that cause B cells to be overactive and respond in detrimental ways to some viruses and bacteria. Epidemiology studies showed that the

* These include inhibitors of Bruton's tyrosine kinase, phosphodiesterase, and other monoclonal antibodies that target B cells.

Epstein-Barr virus (EBV), acting in concert with this genetic predisposition, is a prime suspect.* EBV living inside B cells might be instructing the immune system to attack the brain's myelin insulation because the structure of some EBV protein fragments resembles those of brain proteins.

But other infectious organisms,† not only EBV, can also set off similar misdirected immune responses from high-strung B cells that could lead to MS. So a treatment to definitively cure MS will likely need to target many different B cells, and not only those in the bloodstream but also in other sites such as the surface of the brain.

These are all challenges that can be met. For the first time, we understand the basic mechanisms behind this disease and how the immune system injures the brain. And the knowledge has come not just from the lab, and not just from the bedside. It required bringing the two worlds together—basic research and clinical medicine.

* * *

Adoption of B cell therapy is massive. Patients in more than 100 countries are receiving ocrelizumab, and rituximab, despite never receiving official approval from any regulatory body, is the most commonly used drug for MS in many parts of the world. Clinical studies of analogous monoclonal antibodies‡ show similar stupendous results, and other copycats are likely to follow. For the marketers, lobbyists, and politicians, MS is now a poster child for the promise of biomedical research. The pharmaceutical industry blankets the airways with the message of miracle drugs that they bring to the marketplace. Even the

---

* This is the same virus that causes infectious mononucleosis.

† Other likely triggers are bacteria that live in our gut, including a bug called *Akkermansia*.

‡ Such as ofatumumab and ublituximab.

federal government gets in on the act, touting advances against MS made possible through public investment in medical research.

* * *

Advances in medicine are team efforts. So many physicians and scientists have been part of this odyssey, starting in the early days when cyclophosphamide was first being tested against MS. The insights and contributions of colleagues over the decades were essential for success. The seeds for the next discovery seemed always to be at hand, from young trainees with critical insights, from partners down the hall, from colleagues around the world, all people with the courage to ignore conventional wisdom and join me on a journey that led to a new concept of disease and a life-changing treatment.

I owe an enormous debt of gratitude to my patients, whose trust, strength, and tenacity have been a constant source of inspiration. So many now have opportunities to take charge of their lives and prevent MS from seizing control. The battle is not yet won, but all of the pieces are in place to soon reach the finish line—a cure for MS. The future is filled with promise.

Acknowledgments

My original plan was to write a story of a medical discovery, with the backstory described in just enough detail to appeal to the curious lay reader. As simple as possible, but not simpler than that. I'd be an anonymous witness to the events, and would include elements of autobiography only when absolutely necessary to bring them to life.

During the course of the project, however, the narrative evolved to include a fuller story of my life and career. By introducing the scientist first, I hoped that the science would be even more alive and engaging. Indeed, my personal journey has taken a number of astonishing turns, and these have been great fun to revisit. I also knew that I had an ace up my sleeve—my fascinating, eccentric relatives. Nothing garden variety about them. So I focused on them as much, or more, as I did on myself. And as the story took shape, it spilled over in style, with stops along side roads that were not on any outline or conscious workplan. The writing seemed to take on a mind of its own. This was another unexpected joy; I found myself looking forward to seeing what would happen next.

I've tried to recount the events not only from my perspective but also from those of loved ones, colleagues, patients, and friends whom I've had the good fortune to spend time with along the way. I thank them for agreeing to interviews, endless questions, and requests for documents or old photos, all threads in the quilt that has resulted. The chance to look back has been a gift, increasing even more my appreciation for family members who set me on the road, mentors who could see where the field was headed and provided guidance at key moments, and colleagues who walked the walk with me.

I'm especially thankful to the foundations and private individuals who believed in and supported my work over the years. I've already mentioned the irreplaceable role of the National Multiple Sclerosis Society. After my move from Boston to San Francisco, the Nancy Davis Foundation provided much-needed funding and facilitated new collaborations that strengthened the MS community. And for nearly two decades, the Valhalla Foundation has been beyond generous to our cause; they seemed always to be there whenever help was needed. I owe an enormous debt of thanks to them, and to the scores of private donors, large and small, who shared the vision that MS could be conquered through research.

But my greatest measure of gratitude goes to my patients, whose stories illuminated truths that could otherwise never have been revealed. I owe my education more to them than to any teacher or book.

Discussions with my family, especially my mom Elaine, my brother David, my Uncle Sandy and his wife Sandra, and my sons Stewart, William, and Bennett were great fun and also eye-opening. They helped jog my memories of early life and prompted me to remember how I, and we, felt long ago.

Huge thanks also to my colleagues who put up with many requests to help bring events surrounding MS discoveries into sharper focus: Sunil Agarwal, Andrew Barnecut, Paul Brunetta, Andrew Chan, Peter Chin, Paul Frohna, Hideki Garran, Robert Glanzman, Douglas Goodin, Ludwig Kappos, David Leppert, Marion Letvin, Carl Leventhal, Michelle Libonati, Robin

Lincoln, Fred Lublin, John Marler, Luca Massacesi, Amy Nader, Jorge Oksenberg, Michael Racke, William Rastetter, John Richert, Richard Rudick, Craig Smith, Dan Traficante, Christian Von Buedingen, Howard Weiner, and Shannon Warto. They all helped me to relive the past, and I loved every minute of it. Thanks also to Sam Barondes and Luanne Brizendine for their wise counsel that helped shape the book at critical points.

For the parts that work I can credit the guidance of fantastic editors who brought different things to the table. Amy Hertz encouraged me to write whatever was on the top of my mind that day, but to write every day, fully expecting that 95 percent will be discarded. Thanks to Amy, I had content. Alan Rinzler conceptualized the project as a memoir, creating a structure that brought the tangled threads together into a more or less linear narrative, and even encouraged the intrusions of doo-wop and wrestling. Tim Bartlett at St. Martin's brilliantly edited the manuscript, helping to connect the strands of stories and propel the momentum forward. And special thanks to my agent Sara Camilli, whose wellspring of optimism, energy, and advocacy ensured that we'd reach the finish line. What good fortune to have worked with experts who believed in the project and were generous enough to guide it through to completion.

But no person meant more to this book than my closest friend, my wife Elizabeth Robbins. She was my compass and most diligent editor, wise counselor and masterful problem solver. I'd have never reached the finish line without her. I still don't know how she found time to assist me while also juggling so many other things: caring for the sickest kids imaginable as an oncologist to children with lymphoma and leukemia; serving as mayor of our small town in Marin County; helping to lead a campaign to save a beloved local mountain and hiking trail from developers; caring for kids and grandkids; and still, somehow, finding time to make sure that I was healthy and well-fed. Elizabeth is an astounding force for good, and I cherish the day, more than 40 years ago, when I walked out of the elevator at Harvard's Fernald State Hospital and saw her for the first time. She'd been waiting for me to arrive. I was late as usual . . . and her hair was still damp from that perilous swim far off the coast at Revere Beach.

For me, the process of revisiting the events of a long journey to develop a treatment for MS has been exhilarating, wistful, and also sobering.

Exhilarating, because of the great moments, huge in significance, that marked the major steps forward in the discovery. The breakthrough events. Creating the first real model for MS in the laboratory; the completely unexpected discovery that B cells were at the center of tissue damage in the brain; and the moment when the almost incomprehensible benefits of our therapy were unveiled for the first time. Each was a life-affirming and life-altering experience.

Wistful, to be brought back to those times populated with friends and colleagues, and especially to return, almost as a ghost, to days when I and my loved ones were younger than we are now. Each return reminded me of how wonderful they all were, and are, and how fortunate I've been.

And sobering, because I know all too well that it was a miracle that we were able to stay on course. The MS program could have been killed at many points along the way. At key junctures we were rescued by philanthropists who believed in the value of what we were doing, by industry leaders who took big risks that could never have happened in government or academia, and by simple good luck that, at times, seemed so unlikely as to be preposterous.

All in all, quite a journey.

Index